The New
Hypnosis

The New Hypnosis

By
DANIEL L. ARAOZ, Ed.D.

Professor of Community Mental Health Counseling,
C.W. Post Center of Long Island University,
New York

BRUNNER/MAZEL, *Publishers* • New York

Library of Congress Cataloging in Publication Data

Araoz, Daniel L., 1930–
  The new hypnosis.

  Bibliography: p.
  Includes index.
  1. Hypnotism—Therapeutic use. 2. Hypnotism.
I. Title. [DNLM: 1. Hypnosis. WA 415 A662n]
RC495.A73 1985   615.8′512   84-29327
ISBN 0-87630-387-4

10 9 8 7 6 5 4 3 2

Published by
Brunner/Mazel, Inc.
19 Union Square West
New York, New York 10003

MANUFACTURED IN THE UNITED STATES OF AMERICA

To my sister, Mechy,
and my brothers,
Jorge, Alejandro, and Fernando

Pure logical thinking cannot yield us any knowledge of the empirical world; all knowledge of reality starts from experience and ends in it.

Albert Einstein*

*_Albert Einstein: Philosopher-Scientist_. Copyright by The Library of Living Philosophers, Inc., 1959.

Contents

Foreword

by Ernest L. Rossi, Ph.D.

Renaissance! Renaissance! Hypnosis is once again in an exciting growth phase of its never-ending cycle of self-regeneration. Araoz is a passionate advocate and synthesizer of the current renaissance of hypnosis. In this up-to-date volume, he brings together the scattered skeins of the many apparently conflicting trends in historical and modern hypnosis and weaves them into a tapestry of unity and understanding. He integrates the clinical skills and innovative hypnotherapy of Milton H. Erickson with the academic and experimental work of T. X. Barber, Sarbin and Coe, Ernest Hilgard, and many others in surprising ways. Different approaches from many creative directions are the source of what Araoz calls the "New Hypnosis." They range in application from the psychophysiological (e.g., psychoneuroimmunology) to family therapy and beyond.

What is the New Hypnosis? So vital and enterprising are its practitioners at the present moment that each would see it somewhat differently. Araoz deals with the main issues in a manner that most would agree with, however. Above all, the New Hypnosis is not programming! We have given up the primitive myth of hypnosis as dependent upon a trait called "hypnotizability" which presumed that subjects were somehow rendered into a blank, automaton-like state in which they could be commanded into health. Rather, the New Hypnosis uses the person's own natural mental processes and individuality. Its ideal is to facilitate the process by which people learn to activate their own unique resources and potentials to resolve their own problems in their own ways.

Hypnosis has long been recognized as the mother of the psychotherapies. Both Freud and Jung acknowledged their early use of it. They both evolved new techniques from the rather primitive forms of direct hypnosis they were taught. Freud called his technique "free association" and Jung called his "active imagination." Both thought they were leaving hypnosis behind. Actually, in historical perspective we can now appreciate how free association and active imagination are what Milton H. Erickson would have called indirect forms of hypnosis. The New Hypnosis embraces all approaches that shift the contents of consciousness out of their everyday, conditioned, and limited frames of reference. Free association, active imagination, and all their variations are mind-set altering techniques for freeing the person from the limits of the ordinary to experience the new and creative that is struggling to assert itself. A case could be made for the view that most schools of psychotherapy—including the client-centered approaches, Gestalt, transactional analysis, rational-emotive, behavioral, cognitive, humanistic, existential, and transpersonal—developed from insights that derived from their differing approaches to altering mind-sets. This focus on altering limited mind-sets is the common denominator and the essence of the New Hypnosis.

In this volume it sometimes seems as if the New Hypnosis is in the position of a distraught mother who calls back all her lost psychotherapeutic children, who have been wandering in the wilderness of an uncomprehending world, and struggles to unite them into a fractious but fecund family. It will never happen, but Araoz makes a commendable effort to demonstrate its plausibility and usefulness.

The boon and bane of the New Hypnosis lie in the new insights and skills that are required of the hypnotherapist. The new observational and communication skills that it emphasizes are a boon to the therapist who seeks to awaken from her/his dogmatic slumbers of the traditional teachings of the past. The challenge of learning the New Hypnosis will heighten the awareness and competence of all therapists, whatever their previous level of training or school of thought. The bane of the New Hypnosis, however, is that we may become so overwhelmed by this explosion of innovation that we will be tempted to take the easy route: that of dogmatizing those few approaches we do manage to learn and shutting out the rest before we thoroughly understand the entire scope of the new field and consolidate it with empirical research.

It has been exactly a dozen years since I began my studies with Milton H. Erickson as my personal route to the New Hypnosis. These years have not been easy. To give up the deeply ingrained assumptions of my academic training in early learning theory and behaviorism, and my later training in Freudian and Jungian analysis, was continually disturbing and at times disheartening. To learn to use such radically new approaches as paradoxical intervention, implication, double binds, symptom prescription, and reframing via second-order or metalevel realities kept me in conceptual vertigo for quite some time. Again and again I have been forced to outgrow the childhood of yesterday's understanding. Even today I must struggle to work through my learned limitations to achieve better levels of therapeutic understanding and functioning.

Thus, while Araoz's presentation of the New Hypnosis is exhilarating at times, we must carefully acknowledge that it will require serious effort on our part to integrate it with integrity. On a personal level it requires an open acknowledgment of our need to continually reawaken to further growth in our understanding and skills. On a professional level it requires the humility to recognize the still limited horizons of our verified knowledge and the need to support and expand the empirical-experimental research required to substantiate and extend what we can only believe we now know.

Los Angeles, CA

Preface

by Theodore Xenophon Barber, Ph.D.

During the past 30 years dramatic changes have occurred in the way hypnosuggestive procedures are used in psychotherapy. The client-centered hypnosuggestive approaches that characterize the 1980s are much more resilient, permissive, and collaborative than the hypnotist-centered approaches, focusing on ritualistic hypnotic induction procedures and direct suggestions, which were still dominant in the 1950s. These marked changes that have occurred in one generation are due mainly to three important sets of events.

First of all, the new hypnosuggestive procedures have been stimulated by the results of the in-depth research in hypnosis that took place in the late 50s, 60s, and 70s, and is continuing, at a somewhat reduced pace, in the 80s. During this period, the Federal Government of the United States, especially the National Institutes of Health, poured at least five million dollars into research in hypnosis. Major laboratories were established by Hilgard, Orne, and Barber, and roughly 1,000 scientific papers casting a new light on virtually all aspects of hypnosis were published by these and other researchers, such as Weitzenhoffer, Spanos, Shor, Sheehan, Sarbin, Perry, Levitt, Fromm, Evans, Edmonston, Coe, and Bowers.

Although these active investigators disagreed on secondary issues, a general consensus was reached that hypnosis had been seriously misconceived and misrepresented and was *not* what it was generally thought to be. For over a century, the belief that was accepted by the general public, and that was not vigorously challenged by the authorities in the field, was that, when highly trained hypnotists had completed their induction procedures with cooperative subjects, virtually all of the subjects were in a state of hypnosis or trance in which they had either lost the ability or could not make the effort to initiate their own cognitions and behaviors and, consequently, their thoughts, experiences, and behaviors could be guided by the hypnotist.

Although this rigid conception is still prevalent among the public at large, it is not accepted by any serious present-day researcher in hypnosis. Instead, there is a consensus among researchers that how individuals respond to hypnosuggestions, e.g., to suggestions for deep relaxation, suggestions for altered sensory experiences such as hand warmth, and suggestions for enhanced strength and endurance, depends far less than had previously been supposed on the hypnotist's formal or ritualistic trance induction procedures and far more on many other complexly interrelated variables, most of which pertain to the subject rather than the hypnotist. These interacting variables which determine responsiveness include: the subject's expectancies and beliefs about hypnosis; the subject's attitudes and motivations towards the specific situation; the subject's preexisting abilities to imagine, to fantasize, to daydream, and to have natural, hypnotic-like experiences in daily life; the subject's feelings towards, beliefs about, and interpersonal relationship with the hypnotist; and the hypnotist's "communicative potency," that is, his or her ability to present ideas or suggestions that are personally meaningful and profound for the particular subject.

The shift from the hypnotist-centered, rather authoritarian approaches of the 50s to the client-centered, more democratic approaches of the 80s was also stimulated by changes in American culture that were occurring during this time. These cultural changes included: a marked increase in the average educational level of Americans; a significant expansion of information sources, especially television; and an increasing awareness among large segments of the population of unnecessary and continuous military involvements, as well as the constant threat of nuclear holocaust leading to protest movements and a greater readiness to challenge existing authorities. As the American culture changed during the 50s, 60s, and 70s, traditional hypnotist-centered procedures, which focused on ritualistic trance induction procedures and on authoritarian suggestions, seemed increasingly outdated, quaint, and even foreign to more and more therapists and their clients.

A third important factor that underlies the new hypnosuggestive approaches is the development of psychotherapy that has occurred during the past 30 years. During this period many innovative psychotherapeutic approaches were developed that tended to be more resilient, creative, permissive, democratic, and collaborative than earlier psychotherapies. Innovative psychotherapeutic approaches such as client-centered therapy, Gestalt therapy, existential therapy, cognitive-behavior therapy, and humanistic therapy, which either did not exist or were new in the 50s, became part of the armamentarium of the creative therapist of the 80s. Since the new hypnosuggestive procedures were developed at the same time as these more flexible and permissive psychotherapeutic approaches, and since the hypnosuggestive methods and the psychotherapeutic approaches, were used together by the same therapist and had to be harmonious and congruent with each other, the new hypnosuggestive methods also tended to be more resilient, creative, permissive, and collaborative. Thus, during this period, both the hypnosuggestive procedures and the more general psychotherapeutic approaches utilized by such innovators as Erickson, Sacerdote, Spiegel, and Watkins became less ritualistic and more client-centered. In fact, very early during this period Erickson began to shift increasingly to client-centered approaches that not only markedly influenced the development of hypnosuggestive procedures but also affected the development of psychotherapy in general.

This useful book by Araoz continues the forward movement of the "new hypnosis." It codifies basic principles and presents helpful examples of their implementation. It clarifies the role of the hypnosuggestive therapist as a teacher or guide, forming permissive and collaborative relations with clients, and helping them to feel, imagine, think, and experience in new ways. It appropriately emphasizes the importance of hypnosuggestive therapists being fully involved with their clients and communicating with them ("giving suggestions") not just in a verbal, intellectual way but with feelings, emotions, involvement, and commitment.

When using the "old hypnosis," therapists typically administered formal and often ritualistic trance induction procedures, tested the patient for "trance depth," and were bothered and concerned if they thought the patient was not sufficiently "hypnotized." Therapists utilizing the new hypnosuggestive procedures are aware of the fallacious assumptions underlying the concern with "trance depth," and, as Araoz points out, they emphasize helping the client learn new skills in utilizing hypnosuggestions for peace of mind, tranquility, and self-improvement. Since the aim is to guide clients to become aware of and to stop their automatic negative self-suggestions while simultaneously learning to use constructive suggestions, there is much more emphasis now on teaching the client a new kind of self-hypnosis involving a calm and focused mental rehearsal of the skills, attitudes, and ways of being that the client is aiming to attain. This approach has implications far beyond the closed therapeutic setting. Viewed from the perspective that Araoz presents in this text, the New Hypnosis teaches us all to use self-hypnotic rehearsals to attain peace of mind and to function with more focused awareness and proficiency in our daily lives. This book thus points the way to an improvement in our therapeutic skills and also to improvement in the lives of both ourselves and our clients.

Framingham, MA

Introduction

The first chapter in my book, *Hypnosis and Sex Therapy* (1982), was titled "The New Hypnosis." Several people whose professionalism I respect suggested that I expand on that chapter and its concepts. Thinking about it, I realized that the New Hypnosis is a reality, especially in the last 10–15 years in the English-speaking world, as Chapter 1 will explain.

This book is a presentation of a most effective method to help people reach goals which, though desired, seemed to be unattainable previously. This method is designated as the New Hypnosis because it is rooted in concepts and principles associated with scientific hypnosis, as documented since the time of Mesmer (circa 1775). The New Hypnosis reaches beyond the scope of traditional hypnosis, on the one hand, and beyond the rather narrow focus of the so-called Ericksonian hypnosis with its offshoots, such as Neurolinguistic Programming, on the other.

The New Hypnosis expands the effectiveness of traditional hypnosis by being more experiential, more client-centered, and less tied up with experimental concepts carried over from the laboratory. It also integrates purely clinical applications of hypnosis, as most of the published work of Erickson does (see Gibson, 1984), with the evidence gathered by T. X. Barber and his associates (see References) on the effectiveness of the nontraditional use of clinical hypnosis.

I do not equate the New Hypnosis with the Ericksonian approaches to hypnosis. Initially I had planned on adding a subtitle to the book, "In the footsteps of Milton H. Erickson," as one of my workshops has been announced in several parts of this country. Then, the growing cultism developing around Erickson from coast to coast in the United States of America and even abroad became a serious concern. I did not want to be part of the Milton H. Erickson cult because cultism is self-limiting. Erickson taught something much greater than his personal work using his idiosyncrasies and humor, his unorthodox methods and parables. Some now try to mimic him to the point of sounding like him (the *old* Milton, mind you!), repeating his anecdotes as if they had sacramental value, using paradox just because it sounds more like Erickson (or rather, *Milton*). Cultism is a common inconvenience of all great masters, in religion and philosophy as well as in psychotherapy.

But the cultists miss the point of Erickson's legacy. His work taught us that the therapist has to focus attentively and totally on the client's needs and experiences of the moment. Only within that framework can the therapist be himself* and adapt his approach accordingly. The Ericksonian cult contradicts his main teaching.

The New Hypnosis owes much to Erickson, however. But it is much more than Ericksonian, embracing elements of many researchers and clinicians within the field of traditional hypnosis. It also builds on theoretical and methodological elements of existential/humanistic psychotherapy, on cognitive/behavior therapy, and on awareness/experiential therapy. Finally, the New Hypnosis develops out of the research done outside the field of traditional hypnosis in the areas of imagination, brain bilaterality, and human change, with its many ramifications into values theory, perception, and world image.

Although the theoretical foundation is important to justify and validate the New Hypnosis, this book is primarily practical and oriented to clinical use in psychotherapy. However, this does not

---

*In order to avoid sexist language, I have used the plural whenever possible. However, in cases where this became cumbersome, I interchange masculine and feminine pronouns. I ask the reader's indulgence.

mean that it is a clinical recipe book, listing "how-to" techniques of therapy. On the contrary, it aims at promoting the *understanding* of the principles of the New Hypnosis so that the practicing mental health professional can justify the rules for effective human change proposed herein. Nevertheless, how *to apply* these principles and rules is the ultimate purpose of this book, so that mental health workers may develop successfully *their own* ingenuity and creativity, their sensitive awareness of the client's current reality, and their adaptive health-enhancing skills in any given situation with all its unique human circumstances—biological, cultural and social, psychological, and spiritual. If psychotherapy is a method to activate a person's own psychological healing forces, the sooner this method is learned the healthier the person will be. Because of this belief, the book is written with the motivated client in mind, as will be explained below.

The book is also concerned with the mental health practitioner's *awareness* of his clients, so that his interventions are truly successful. Achievement of goals and economy of time and energy are primary concerns for most therapists. However, the controversy between insight therapy and other, more experiential interventions is far from settled. This famous "gap" in all insight therapy is at the crux of the debate. This gap is the connection between intellectual insight and the personal *experience* of real change. Actually, the argument even questions the very necessity of intellectual insight. This is not the place to rekindle the old controversy but simply to mention it in connection with effective therapy. The evidence we have at present is a strong justification for the New Hypnosis as a powerful way to help people change freely and deeply.

That the origin of people's change is an inner experience rather than a reasoned conviction is quite factual from what we observe in many aspects of human behavior: from religious conversions and career changes to divorces and drastic alterations in longstanding habits such as smoking, overdrinking, and overeating. Studying carefully the position held by the Nancy school of hypnosis (especially the so-called New Nancy school), we find that much of what they understood by suggestion and autosuggestion falls under the concept of inner experiences, as opposed to intellectual insight or reasoned convictions. For example, it is interesting to remember that what the Nancy school defended with its "Laws of Suggestion" fits neatly with current data on the bilaterality of the human brain.* Their distinction between *will* and *imagination* refers, unknowingly, to left- and right-hemispheric activities. Quotes from Coué, such as "The will must not intervene in the practice of autosuggestion" or "We get unsatisfactory results when we aim at the reeducation of the will. What we have to work for is the reeducation of the imagination," become more meaningful to us if we translate them in modern bilaterality terms.

Because of this underlying link with the New Nancy school, the designation of the *New* Hypnosis seems more appropriate than others, such as *modern, naturalistic, Ericksonian,* or *indirect. New* also reflects the goal of the approach described in this book, namely, human change, newness—which is the purpose, at least theoretically, of any form of psychotherapy. But because *human* change follows definite laws related to right-hemispheric functioning, *hypnosis* is kept in the title, even though many traditional hypnotists will strongly disagree with my understanding of hypnosis. From the evidence accumulated in the last decade or so, it is now irrefutable that hypnosis is related to right-hemispheric functioning. However, hypnosis may be taken in a much wider sense than by the traditionalists to include all mental activities which bypass left-hemispheric functioning, whether induced or spontaneous.

The New Hypnosis has applications in all areas of human

---

*The use of cerebral hemispheric language throughout the book is purely didactic and almost metaphorical; one must be fully cognizant of its limitations and even dangers. The limitations arise from the many details science is still discovering about the functioning of the human brain and especially the integration of left- and right-hemispheric activities. The dangers of using bilaterality concepts in trying to explain hypnotic realities lie in oversimplification, as if we had the answer to complex and intricate questions which only future research will be able to provide.

A sober presentation of hemispheric bilaterality in the human brain is offered by Watzlawick (1978), who explains the concept as a heuristic device and presents the experimental evidence to justify its use.

change. Thus, this book does not restrict itself to individual therapy but covers the value of the New Hypnosis in family therapy and even in what may be called self-development or personal growth. People will benefit from learning to use their minds and avoid negative self-hypnosis (Araoz, 1981). In this sense of teaching people, from childhood on, the value of constructive and positive suggestions to be used in all human endeavors, *education* is a natural area for the New Hypnosis. From the earliest contributions of the Nancy school, the "general application of the doctrine of suggestion," as Bernheim called it in 1887, has included education. Baudouin, another important figure in the New Nancy school, devotes a chapter of his book originally published in 1913 to "Suggestion in the Education of Children." Nowadays we would talk about a self-help approach. The point is that people can learn to use self-hypnosis to improve their lives. This trend appeared for a while among traditionalists as well (Le Cron with his books on self-hypnosis is a good example), but was overpowered by the more general trend of heterohypnosis. This resulted in shifting the focus from "education" to psychotherapy; from viewing hypnosis as a practical method for self-improvement, easily learned by any normal individual, to viewing it as a highly specialized "medical" technique, dangerous when not used under direct professional supervision.

The New Hypnosis, among other things, reverses the trend. It returns this mental skill (not *trait*) to the hands of all well-motivated normal people who want to learn how to use it for their self-improvement. Hypnosis *can be learned* by "the common man" without regard to the so-called hypnotizability trait. Indeed, regular use of hypnosis would benefit individuals and society greatly. The benefits form a long list, from greater self-confidence and self-esteem to increased inner peace of mind. Tapping our inner resources, we find several positive rewards, such as a different world image than the one progressively formed from neurotic needs through the years. This more realistic view of the world usually leads to a resolution of angry and violent feelings, which, if shared by many, will benefit society and interpersonal living.

The New Hypnosis, then, is not just a method of therapy. As

a concept it comprises an attitude, a willingness to recognize in a practical way the influence of the inner mind—the subconscious —in every aspect of a person's life, and an effort to learn how to use that influence of the subconscious to the best advantage. My advice to students interested in these techniques is to first experience them in themselves. Only after we become convinced from the results we notice in our lives that the New Hypnosis is valuable will we be able to use it successfully with others.

This book hopes to help in the discovery of the New Hypnosis by being a guide for this unexplored territory. The only requirement to benefit from it is to approach it with an open mind, realizing that the New Hypnosis fits comfortably in any form of psychotherapy and human communication. It is not a different school—we know we have too many schools and gurus already; rather, it is a method to be applied by anyone interested in making psychotherapy and human interaction more effective.

Acknowledgments

It would be impossible to express gratitude to all the teachers who have contributed to the shaping of my thinking, from Augustine of Hippo and Thomas Aquinas to Rogers, Ellis, Lazarus, and Watzlawick. The innumerable authors, colleagues, and teachers to whom I am indebted are buried someplace in the recesses of my memory and would form a long procession. I know that without them I would not be who I am today. My humble thanks are a constant in my daily life.

To those nearer, I feel the need to express my gratitude and indebtedness: my friends, Jerry Kushel and Ed Debus, whose stimulating conversations always generate an energy and vitality leading to new horizons; and my children, Lee and Nadine, who even through the difficult times of their parents' separation and divorce, gave me courage and "ánimo," as we say in Spanish ("soul" is an incomplete translation, but is close), and put up with my long hours of writing with an understanding and maturity beyond their years. My typist, Joanne Potratz, has been much more than just that. She became an editor, advisor, and coach— and I am very grateful. Last but not least, I want to mention Angela Vitale. She not only helped me with the references, editing, and organization of the book and typing certain segments of it; she also admonished me, taught me, and helped me. Without her, the last few weeks of writing would have been impossible and the book would never have been finished.

Finally, I want to express my deepest gratitude to those who

taught me most of what I know about psychotherapy and hypnosis, to those who made it possible for me to make the synthesis I call the New Hypnosis—namely, the many clients I've seen
in the last 25 years of practice.

"Gracias" in Spanish is a way of asking for a blessing—God's
graces—on those who have been good to us. To all these good
people I say "Gracias!"

Part I

Validation

This part comprises three chapters which attempt to present the evidence, both historical and theoretical, for the New Hypnosis. The third chapter, however, is already an overview of clinical techniques which fit into the general approach explained in this book. For those who are familiar with the traditional method of hypnosis and also for those who, being psychotherapists, want to learn hypnosis to enrich their work, these three chapters provide the "justification" needed to try a new approach. The 12 techniques listed in Chapter 3 indicate the wealth of methods available to the psychotherapist who intends to employ this novel form of psychotherapy.

1

The Influence of
the New Nancy School

By placing the New Hypnosis in historical perspective I intend to connect it with a fairly established tradition in mental health. Starting in inverse chronological order we find T. X. Barber (1983) currently referring to hypnosuggestions or hypnosuggestive techniques. Basing his approach on careful research, as is his style, Barber is echoing the words attributed to Bernheim by Baudouin (1922), "There is no hypnotism, there is only suggestion," and Coué's later statement, "There is no suggestion, there is only self-suggestion." The New Nancy school, as represented by Baudouin, discovered the dynamics and rules of self-suggestion. T. X. Barber has collected data and conducted his own experimental and clinical studies clarifying the New Nancy school's teachings and refining our practical understanding of suggestion.

THE TEACHINGS OF THE NEW NANCY SCHOOL (CA. 1920)

The New Hypnosis is connected with the Nancy school, which moved away from the Salpêtrière school (Araoz, 1982a), contrary to the direction Traditional Hypnosis and psychiatry have taken. Though there were many famous figures at Nancy, it is possible to view Liébeault and Bernheim as the founders of the *school* (meaning, of course, the teachings propounded by the group, rather than an academic setting), while Coué acts as a bridge to the New Nancy school, of which Baudouin is the best known exponent. This school flourished from the second half of the 19th century well into the early 1930s. From what I understand, the designation of "New" appears when the Nancy school refused to continue the controversy with the Salpêtrière and took the focus of attention away from hypnosis and onto suggestion. Just as hypnotism had become separated from mysticism and the occult by Braid in Scotland and Bertrand in France, suggestion became dissociated from hypnotism by Coué and his disciple Baudouin. Both held that hypnosis was one manifestation of *the effect of imagination and self-suggestion* on a person's perceptions, moods, behavior, and even physiological functions. This idea is still unacceptable in many circles, especially the medical establishment, in spite of the mounting evidence that *nonconscious self-suggestions are an important variable in human suffering, both mental* (Araoz, 1981; Blumenthal, 1984) *and physical* (T. X. Barber, 1981b; Hall, 1983; Holden, 1978).

An attempt to summarize the position of the New Nancy school runs the risk of producing an incomplete and unfair statement. However, the core of their finding—that willpower and effort are unable to produce effective change—agrees admirably with later findings on the bilaterality of the human brain. The school's basic tenet can be translated into modern terms: Effective change is brought about experientially through right-hemispheric activity, rather than through reason and logic (left-hemispheric functioning).

The three essential contributions of the New Nancy school may be listed as follows: First, and to repeat, it is not *will* (left-hemispheric functioning) that produces change but *imagination* (right-hemispheric activity). Their famous "law of reversed effect" states that conscious effort of the will is useless as long as the imagination is adverse to that effort. The second teaching stresses *self-*suggestion. Hetero-suggestions work only when they echo what the individuals are suggesting to themselves in truth. An important corollary of this is the deemphasis of the hypnotist-as-therapist, who becomes, rather, a teacher or guide with whose help the individual learns to use self-suggestion effectively. Finally, the third feature of the New Nancy school is that self-suggestion operates at the level of nonconscious thinking or what we would now understand as experiential, right-hemispheric thinking. Therefore, the task at hand is to use the nonconscious mode of thinking, or to engage the right hemisphere, initially bypassing conscious thinking.

Underlying these three points is the uninhibited emphasis of the New Nancy school on the educational applications of these teachings. The emphasis moved from clinical (hypnotist–client) to that of personal enrichment, a logical consequence of the insistence on *self*-suggestions.

Self-suggestion is the Key

Any thought, belief, mental impression, or image can act as a self-suggestion affecting perception, mood, and behavior. In cases of either mental, behavioral, or even physical dysfunction, nonconscious self-suggestions of a negative nature are at work, as T. X. Barber (1979a; 1981a, b; 1982a; 1984b) has demonstrated. But, according to Baudouin's (1922) succinct principle, "Whatever suggestion has done, suggestion can undo." The challenge, then, is to learn to use suggestions in a constructive, effective, ego- and health-enhancing way.

Experiential Thinking

This brings us back to T. X. Barber, for whom the essence of hypnosis is *not* the practice of the *external maneuvers* commonly associated with hypnosis. These include induction, physical passivity, the hypnotist directing the cognitive process of the subject or client, and mental (e.g., amnesia or hallucinations) or physical (e.g., catalepsy) "hypnotic" phenomena or outcomes deemed to result from the entire hypnotic induction. For Barber (1984a) the essence of hypnosis is the effect of communications (sugges-

tions) 1) to let go of extraneous concerns and 2) to feel—remember
—imagine—experience in new or unusual ways. It should be kept
in mind that responsiveness to suggestions has usually been seen
as the major goal of hypnosis. Both the traditional scales of hypnotic responsiveness and the concern with depth of hypnosis depend on the subject's responsiveness to the suggestions given.
If subjects responded to suggestions, hypnosis was achieved; if
they did not, there was no hypnosis.

T. X. Barber (1978; 1981) has reviewed close to 100 reports,
studies, and cases analyzing the effects of suggestions on bodily
processes and healing, coming to the bold conclusion that ideas
can affect the physiological activities of the cells in the human
body (1984a). Semantic input is decoded as somatic output. In
Chapter 7 I will discuss at greater length the effects of suggestions on bodily processes.

In the area of psychological effects, T. X. Barber (1979a; 1984b;
in press) also gives us a comprehensive review of the evidence.
His analysis is helpful in pointing out the confusion originated
by considering "good" hypnotic subjects as the only ones who
could benefit from hypnosis. According to T. X. Barber, good
or talented hypnotic subjects are those who have generally had
more life-time practice in imagining, in retrieving past experiences
and feelings (while fantasizing), and in putting aside other concerns by becoming deeply absorbed in fantasy.

Unwittingly, Traditional Hypnosis, with its reliance on such
measurement instruments as the Stanford Hypnotic Susceptibility Scales (Weitzenhoffer and Hilgard, 1959, 1962), the Hypnotic
Induction Profile (Spiegel, 1973), or even the Creative Imagination Scale (Barber and Wilson, 1979; Wilson and Barber, 1978),
has given the impression that subjects who score poorly on these
scales are not hypnotizable, i.e., cannot benefit from hypnotic
suggestions. As T. X. Barber (in press) points out, certain suggestions, such as those for amnesia and visual hallucinations, are
easily experienced by good hypnotic subjects, but this type of
suggestion is relatively unimportant in psychotherapeutic work.
He claims that most useful hypnosuggestions are accepted even
by those whose fantasizing ability is not highly developed and

who are not completely detached from reality concerns. These suggestions can become valuable catalysts with most clients as long as the therapist modifies them according to the personality of each client.

As I shall indicate in Chapter 2, J. Barber (1982) makes a useful distinction regarding the use of these traditional scales. He reminds us that what they may really measure is not the ability to benefit from hypnosis but simply the response to direct suggestions.

DIFFERENT TYPES OF SUGGESTIONS

Baudouin (1922) described three types of suggestions: spontaneous, induced, and reflective. Two elements are essential in all three categories: 1) an idea, mental representation, or image accepted by the subject—usually uncritically; and 2) the "transformation" of it into some change, physical or mental, in the subject. "The idea takes on flesh," to echo a Biblical statement, but through a subconscious process. Thus, as Baudouin defines suggestion, it is "the subconscious realization of an idea" (p. 29).

Spontaneous Suggestions

These are everyday occurrences. Advertising works because of suggestions: The item we perceive as attractive becomes something we want to have or do. The idea becomes something in ourselves which we tend to realize without being fully aware of the process. Examples of spontaneous suggestions abound: Knowing that the temperature is low tends to make us feel cold; dealing with someone who is either happy or depressed tends to make us share in that feeling; seeing someone yawn is an invitation for us to yawn, and so on.

To classify all instances of spontaneous self-suggestion, Baudouin distinguishes between representative, affective, motor, and conditional suggestions. A brief example of each is enough for our purposes. In the first category, we find situations where a stimulus triggers a mental representation, as when the sight of a dog may spontaneously initiate images of another dog the individual had a long time ago. The affective category comprises spontaneous self-suggestions of pain, pleasure, or any other feeling elicited by *the idea of a sensation of pleasure, or pain* or any other feeling. The example of yawning, mentioned above, belongs to the motoric spontaneous self-suggestions. Finally, conditional self-suggestions are those situations in which a thing previously connected with something else becomes the stimulus for that "something else." Habits such as drinking coffee and cigarette smoking are examples of conditional self-suggestions. As Baudouin stated: "Every time that so-and-so happens, so-and-so will follow" (1922, p. 121).

Spontaneous self-suggestions are important from our point of view because the same subconscious mechanism which produces undesirable behavior can be learned and directed to work for an individual's benefit and self-enhancement. In this respect, the four laws formulated by the New Nancy school (see Baudouin, 1922, Chapter 10) in its effort to understand how spontaneous self-suggestion operates are to be kept in mind.

The law of concentrated attention affirms that the idea which tends to realize itself is that to which spontaneous attention is given. *The law of auxiliary emotions* states that the emotion accompanying an idea makes it realize itself: the stronger the emotion, the more effective the power of self-suggestion that an idea has.

The law of reversed effort refers to ideas which become subconsciously and spontaneously self-suggestions. All conscious efforts to counteract them are useless and even tend to strengthen the self-suggestion. This is connected with one of the basic principles of the New Hypnosis: conscious, left-hemispheric activity is ineffective in the process of human change. Later, when we discuss reflective self-suggestion, we shall see how to counteract negative spontaneous self-suggestions—what I have called negative self-hypnosis (Araoz, 1981). The law of reverse effort is Coué's main contribution to the New Hypnosis: When the will and the imagination are in conflict, the latter always wins. The more one tries and the more effort or willpower one uses to achieve a personal goal, the less one succeeds. This is why relaxation—the condition in which thoughts can be dealt with gently, peacefully, and nonforcefully—is usually a preliminary to hypnotic change. Goba (1983) bases his hypnotherapeutic approach on this basic principle of nonforceful thinking. He compares the forceful exclusion of unpleasant or disturbing thoughts to a telephone with a hold button:

> An irate caller is on the line with a complaint and you put the caller on hold to gain time to think about your response. By the time you release the hold button you are confronted with the caller's increased frustration due to your delay in dealing with the call. . . . Forceful exclusion of thoughts, like the hold button, may succeed for a while in removing disturbing thoughts from your awareness, but they remain in the unconscious mind waiting, just like the irate caller, to be finally dealt with. (p. 3)

Finally, *the law of subconscious teleology* states that, when a goal has become a self-suggestion, the subconscious finds the means for its attainment. It is easy to apply these laws to several areas which rely on suggestion to attain their ends, such as advertising, education, politics, and persuasion in general. Ideas are presented with attractiveness (first law) and emotional appeal (second law); they are "sold" to us as a very desirable goal, one without which we would not be happy (fourth law) so that all arguments against them are invalid (third law).

Induced Suggestions

These comprise those imposed on us directly from an outside source. The hypnotic suggestions used by both traditional and stage hypnotists fall under this category.

Reflective Suggestions

Reflective suggestions, on the other hand, are what we could designate as constructive, effective, or therapeutic self-hypnosis. These are the self-suggestions we can learn in order to improve our lives, to change for the better, and to choose our destiny. In Baudouin's words: "We have merely to substitute for spontaneous attention that voluntary attention with which, as civilized adults, we are all familiar" (1922, p. 143). If the desired suggestions will come into effect "with the minimum of effort," relaxation provides the best condition. My formula of hypnosis (H = RIS) is a shortcut to remember that *Imagination* and *Suggestions* must be used in a *Relaxed* state.

Reflective suggestions, then, are those thoughts we choose consciously (Blumenthal, 1984) to influence and affect us, but which we assimilate gently, peacefully, in a relaxed state. Or, as T. X. Barber (1984b) has stressed, relaxation in this context mostly means inner peace, tranquility, and calmness, rather than mere muscle relaxation. The aim of any successful psychotherapy is a change for the better, and it seems that reflective self-suggestion is the ultimate mechanism of human change.

Blumenthal (1984) summarizes the effectiveness of this approach in the three steps of what he labels Rational Suggestion Therapy. The first task is to select the "rational" thought which is to substitute for a previously discovered ineffective, self-defeating, "irrational" thought. Let's assume the client has been despondent and depressed since his diagnosis of cancer of the prostate. In the preliminary discussion, the therapist finds that the client is fostering images of complete disability, progressive general deterioration, sexual impotence, and early death with rich details of his wake and funeral. At the same time, the client is repeating to himself several negative statements such as "My life is over," "God is punishing me for my sins," and "I'll never be a man again; I'll be a cripple." At this point, the therapist and the client decide together what "rational" thoughts (statements and images) could be used to substitute for all the above. In this case, thoughts of the health forces at work in the client's body and of the strength of his immune system with detailed imagery (the life energy flowing through the client's body as a powerful river of light, for instance) are chosen. It should be emphasized that these ideas must be truthful.

Then, in the practical phase, the actual self-hypnotic work is done. In a relaxed state, the client is helped to experience in his imagination that powerful life-force at work in his body at that very moment and to repeat to himself such statements as, "My immune system is a strong energy of healing and life," or "I want to allow my health forces to work unimpeded in my body."

The final phase occurs after therapy, when the client practices the above exercise on his own. Subsequent therapy sessions are used to refine and reinforce the effective self-suggestions. As Blumenthal (1984) indicates: "It is desirable to attempt to alter unprofitable autosuggestion with rationally developed autosuggestion in advance of anticipated (negative) conditions. This technique may be used for the immense benefit of the individual whose current ideas are working against his/her own best interests" (p. 3). Drawing on Ellis (1973), Blumenthal underlines the need to aim suggestions at ideas (beliefs, values) rather than behavior or emotion, since the thought is the genesis of emotional and behavioral expression. "If the symptom alone is blocked without a fundamental improvement in the causal idea, that idea will exert influence on another area, seeking to establish a new association of conditions and behaviors, as real and imagined alternatives become available to the individual" (p. 4).

INDEBTEDNESS TO THE NEW NANCY SCHOOL

The New Hypnosis refines and enriches, with the help of recent research evidence, what the New Nancy school taught almost a century ago. This new research draws on current knowledge about the bilaterality of the human brain (Ley and Freeman, 1984), the dynamics of self-suggestion (T. X. Barber, 1979a, b; 1981a, b; 1982a, b; 1983; 1984b; in press), and the alternate ways of using hypnosis (Erickson and Rossi, 1981).

The clinical applications that flow from this approach are vast and even revolutionary. Now we know why most psychotherapy is a waste of time and energy (Eysenck, 1967). What produces human change is not talk, analysis, intellectual awareness—all left-hemispheric activities—but inner experiencing. By activating right-hemispheric functioning a person is able to experience in a new, individualized, and existential way the changes her intellect recognizes as desirable but her emotions (for lack of a better description) refuse to accomplish. Therapists often talk about getting clients in touch with their feelings. The New Hypnosis shows how to do this effectively. We cannot get in touch with feelings by "understanding" them. In order to change, we must experience ourselves differently. Change starts with the new inner perception/experience—what T. X. Barber (1984a) describes as "feeling—remembering—thinking—imagining—experiencing" new inner realities.

The New Nancy school gave us the important information on self-suggestions: Everything that we accept uncritically affects our life—our perception, evaluation, interpretation, and meaning of external or internal realities. This school also gave us the method by which we can use self-suggestions to enrich our lives.

The New Hypnosis teaches us the method by which we *can* change. Departing from the unnecessary rituals of Traditional Hypnosis, we can still utilize the special modality of "thinking," commonly associated with hypnosis. But we are able to do it in more natural, spontaneous ways, with the emphasis on our own learning of how to do it, rather than on the ministrations of an expert. In Erickson's (Erickson, Rossi, and Rossi, 1976) view the New Hypnosis is "the process of evoking and utilizing a patient's own mental processes in ways that are outside his usual range of intentional or voluntary control" (p. 145). Chapter 4 will explain this in more detail: How we know what to look for and what to focus on during the therapy sessions in order to make every minute of therapist-patient interaction count towards change for the better.

In this time of increased consumer demands, of greater dissatisfaction with professional arrogance and pedantry, the New Hypnosis provides an honest and effective method to help the people who come to us for change. *We* don't change them, *we* don't cure them. We teach them how to use inner resources and energy that *they* possess but did not know how to utilize. The New Nancy school emphasized this aspect of learning and self-improvement, calling it the pedagogic aspect of self-suggestion. The New Hypnosis minimizes the clinical, pathology-oriented view of human problems and emotional suffering. In the tradition of existential humanistic psychology (Yalom, 1980), it seeks the strengths and positive aspects of the human condition in order to enhance them and build on them. What Erickson (Erickson, Rossi, and Rossi, 1976) stated about hypnotic phenomena comes to mind: They are not extraordinary happenings; they are experiences which lie hidden and untapped in the human psyche but which can be brought to life, as it were, in order to help people live fuller, more satisfying lives.

CONCLUSION

The New Hypnosis is not a new school of psychotherapy but a systematic method within which any valid psychotherapeutic modality can function. This chapter has reviewed the connection between the New Nancy school and the New Hypnosis. By departing from the traditional accoutrements of hypnosis as it was understood and practiced up until recently (T. X. Barber, 1983, refers to pre-1970 inductions), the New Hypnosis connects with the New Nancy school. This group proposed a modality of hypnosis at about the same time that Traditional Hypnosis, following the Salpêtrière school, started. Historical circumstances beyond our concern in this book made the Traditional Hypnosis popular in psychiatry and clinical psychology, while the Nancy group was dismissed by the medical establishment. But in recent years, thanks mainly to the scientific contributions of T. X. Barber and his students and the clinical innovations of Erickson and his disciples, we are rediscovering the wealth of practical applications derived from the teachings of, first, the Nancy school and, a decade later, the New Nancy school.

It is interesting to note that this trend towards a more natural use of hypnotic techniques is appearing in Europe also (Zeig, 1985), indicating a general retreat from the exaggerated professionalism of the last century or so and a move towards a more responsible, holistic involvement in one's own well-being.

2

The Paradox of
the New Hypnosis

From the point of view of Traditional Hypnosis, there is a paradox in being able to obtain all the benefits of hypnosis without its rituals. It is paradoxical that people are "hypnotized" without induction; that low-scoring subjects in the traditional hypnotizability scales obtain good hypnotic results; that every normal person benefits from hypnosis and that the clinician uses any manifestation of the clients' subconscious mental activity to lead them into the hypnosis experience. Thus, it can be said that the New Hypnosis is "hypnosis without hypnosis," to borrow Kuhner's (1962) phrase.

The roots of the New Hypnosis (Araoz, 1982a,b) are as deep as those of Traditional Hypnosis. Most people, including professionals, are familiar with Traditional Hypnosis, the understanding of which comes closer to that of the Salpêtrière school with Charcot, Janet, and other such giants of psychiatry. But, lately, two important currents have helped crystallize the New Hypnosis. There are the contributions of Milton H. Erickson (Erickson and Rossi, 1975, 1979, 1981; Haley, 1967; Rossi, 1980; Zeig, 1982)

This chapter is adapted from presentations at the Annual Scientific Meetings of the American Society of Clinical Hypnosis in Denver, October 1982, and in Dallas, November 1983.

from a clinical point of view, and of T. X. Barber (1957, 1969, 1978; Barber, Spanos and Chaves, 1974; Wilson and Barber, 1982) from an experimental and scientifically controlled reference point.

Nevertheless, the New Hypnosis is not only the product of these two important figures. Other significant contributions come from studies on cognitive processes (Beck, 1976; De Stefano, 1977; Katz, 1978, 1979; Katz and Crawford, 1978; Meichenbaum, 1974; Spanos, 1971); from research on imagery (J. Barber and Adrian, 1982; Sheikh, 1982; Sheikh and Shaffer, 1979; Singer, 1975; Singer and Pope, 1978); from the discoveries of brain bilaterality (Pribram, 1971; Rossi, 1977; Shulik, 1979; Watzlawick, 1978); and from investigations on the modifications of hypnotic receptivity (Diamond, 1974, 1977a,b; Kinney and Sachs, 1974; Sachs and Anderson, 1967).

Among those writers more specifically in the field of hypnosis could be listed many who have provided insights beneficial to the New Hypnosis. Thus, Shor (1959) developed the concept of hypnosis taking place when the generalized reality orientation is weakened; Miller, Galanter and Pribram (1960) saw the planning function being abandoned in hypnosis, recognizing a gradation in this switch, as Shor had done; Kuhner (1962), from his dental experience, advocated "hypnosis without hypnosis" when it takes place as the natural development in a relationship in which the patient has a need for hypnosis and the therapist provides the conditions to make the experience possible. Fromm's (1977) utilization of primary process thinking and Rossi's (Erickson and Rossi, 1979) depotentiation of left-hemispheric activity in hypnosis helped develop the nontraditional view. Finally, the credit for trying to demystify hypnosis and for viewing it as a natural phenomenon must go to both T. X. Barber (1969) and to Hilgard (1977). The latter's neo-dissociation theory helped explain the naturalness of the hypnotic experience. Elsewhere, I have summarized some of these sources (Araoz, 1982a).

The formulation, understanding, and application of hypnosis emerging from all these directions is different from that of Traditional Hypnosis. The latter stresses (a) the trance state, (b) the operator's induction ritual, and (c) the subject's talent needed to produce the trance state. In contrast, the main concern of the New Hypnosis is with *the process* and *the skills* needed and *to be learned* by the client in order *to enjoy the experience* of hypnosis.

Truly, the New Hypnosis is not new. Only in contrast to what most professionals educated in hypnosis have been taught is it new. And because these professionals practice traditionally, the public also believes that, without the ritualistic paraphernalia and the assessment of hypnotizability and hypnotic depth, there is no hypnosis. The traditional view is also reinforced by entertainers who, for their purpose, dramatize with their antics the magic associated with trance, induction, and hypnotic depth.

The nontraditional conceptualization and use of hypnosis are appropriately called *new* for two main reasons: First is that the New Hypnosis includes the thinking of many modern authors from fields other than hypnosis proper, as mentioned above. Second, to reemphasize, it links the nontraditional approach to the New Nancy school (Baudouin, 1922), as the second generation of clinical researchers following the original group came to be known.

To focus more keenly on the theoretical development leading to the new formulation of hypnosis, Diamond (1978, 1982b) has taken pains to outline the differences between the traditional trance paradigm and what he calls *the cognitive skills model* of hypnosis. This task was begun earlier by T. X. Barber (1972; Barber and Wilson, 1977) who searched for an alternative model for hypnosis following Sarbin's (1962) historical study and theoretical endeavors (Sarbin, 1950; Sarbin and Andersen, 1967; Sarbin and Coe, 1972).

However, perhaps more than anybody else, it was Diamond (1972, 1974, 1977a,b, 1978, 1980, 1983a) who addressed himself to the differences between the old and the new models of hypnosis. In a revised study, he found 30 such differences (Diamond, 1983b). A brief summary would hardly do justice to his important contribution. I must, nevertheless, resign myself to a few comments on Diamond's ideas.

He points to the general agreement about the change in consciousness which occurs in hypnosis. However, what is involved in this altered consciousness is more difficult to define. The traditionalists, according to Diamond (1983b), insist on explaining it in simple terms or on finding a single explanation for the experiential reality of hypnosis, while he analyzes its multidimensional nature. Thus, he starts from the individual's *choice* to modify perceptual experience and follows the person's cognitive alterations employed in order to acquire and experience this altered consciousness. These cognitive processes used by the person in search of the hypnotic experience are imagination and fantasy, enactment, dissociation, distraction, yielding, awareness of body sensations, and so forth. They all have characteristics of *letting go* or giving oneself permission to experience fully whatever comes into awareness.

For many, change is a process from one state to another but always within the known. This is what Watzlawick and colleagues (1974) called first-order change, change within the familiar, change without real surprise. Second-order change is a leap into the unknown, like the urgency to do something heroic or to devote one's life to some subjectively great cause, or like death. In our American culture, falling in love comes close to second-order change in many cases.

There is a paradox in change. If a person changes from one known state to another known state, he really doesn't change. But if he takes the risk of changing from the familiar to the unfamiliar, he steps into the unknown. The change can be so drastic that he ceases to be what he was. This paradox of change was applied to hypnosis by Wick (1983). Effective change occurs when one has an attitude of openness to inner awareness, when one is receptive to experiencing fully what emerges from one's inner self. This receptivity, as Wick explains, is a cognitive process different from both activity and passivity.

But once the person has decided to experience hypnosis—once the person gives himself permission to let go of the ordinary way of thinking—there is an ongoing subtle interplay between voluntary and involuntary behavior, as Diamond (1983b) put it. Reminding us of Hilgard's (1977) research, he notes that even extreme amnesia in hypnosis involves some degree of voluntariness. This is also true of analgesia (Hilgard and Hilgard, 1975), as the discovery of *the hidden observer* reveals. On the other hand, the fact that a person cannot explain how she obtained a specific hypnotic behavior does not necessarily mean that she had no voluntary part in the process. Automatisms fall into this category also. Until there is more evidence, Diamond speculates that "it may well be that while the phenomenologically occurring events are essentially similar, subjects may differ in the ability *to observe* their cognitive processes and, in turn, *to discriminate, utilize and report* such activities" (Diamond, 1983b, p. 15).

What are, then, the essential differences between the two models of hypnosis and the way in which they are used clinically? Before elaborating on these differences I should stress that they are not primarily in the subject's experience of hypnosis, but rather in *the clinician's understanding of the process* (hypnotizability, hypnotic depth, and hetero- vs. self-hypnosis) and in *the techniques used* to both facilitate the experience of hypnosis in the other person and utilize it therapeutically (induction, utilization, and suggestions). Thus, I intend to focus here on these two general topics.

THE UNDERSTANDING OF HYPNOSIS

The New Hypnosis assumes that every normally intelligent and emotionally healthy individual can experience hypnosis (hence the emphasis on self-hypnosis and the disregard for measuring hypnotic depth); and that hypnotizability is at best a fallacious concept derived from laboratory research and dubiously applied in the consulting room.

Hypnotizability

Others have argued powerfully against the alleged universal validity of hypnotizability. J. Barber (1982), for instance, summarizes his comments on this subject by stating: "Our own work [and that of others cited by him] suggests that *what is important in predicting or determining hypnotic responsiveness is* [italics added] not a fixed trait (possibly even genetic) that is measured by a susceptibility test, but *the particular hypnotic approach that is taken with a patient* [italics added] (and perhaps the relationship that develops from this particular approach)" (p. 44). He goes on to distinguish between direct and indirect methods of induction and suggestion, indicating that the latter often work admirably when the former have failed. J. Barber concludes with this interesting thought: "This must tell us that a susceptibility score reflects only responsiveness to a particular hypnotic approach and is not a predictor of general responsivity to hypnosis," as he himself had demonstrated in a previous article on the unhypnotizable (J. Barber, 1980).

If, then, we understand hypnosis as a skill that any normal person can learn rather than a trait, immutable by nature, hypnotizability is not the issue. *The issue is how to apply hypnotic techniques* in order to help an individual benefit from hypnosis.

The skill of hypnosis is a corollary of the human ability to imagine, which means to internally represent sensations belonging to the sensory apparatus of sight, taste, smell, hearing, and kinetic sensations, including skin contact. These internal representations may be within the realm of possibility (I can imagine myself drinking a hot cup of coffee in a cozy log cabin while the wind sweeps a snow-covered landscape outside). They may also be representations of impossible situations (I can imagine myself riding an elephant that is flying over a planet in another galaxy where all people have two heads and only one leg). All normal people use this amazing power of imagination, to the extent that life would be impossible without the ability to reproduce internally things, people, and events experienced externally. Memory seems to be mostly imagination.

When hypnosis is to be used with an individual, the concern of the clinician should not be hypnotizability but the modality of thinking—of reproducing the world internally—that this person prefers or uses comfortably *at the time* (Coe and Sharcoff, 1983). This is easily discovered by the use of language: words, figures of speech, analogies, sentences reflecting mental imagery. By paying attention to the person's language, the clinician will be able to "connect" with the client. In other words, once I realize that this person is now thinking in a more kinetic manner, let's say, than visual or auditory, I can start using kinetic language even though I, personally, may be preferentially visual or auditory.

If imagination is the ability to duplicate internally the world outside—and to embellish it, change it, improve it, or distort it—hypnosis is the ability to so fully immerse oneself in this internal mental activity that the surrounding reality fades away temporarily. T. X. Barber (with Spanos and Chaves, 1974) has argued, for the last 20 years, this point about the importance of imagination as the generic concept to understand hypnosis.

The concept of hypnotizability, therefore, goes to the core of hypnosis. This issue becomes not merely factual, but also philosophical. The New Hypnosis starts with the subject experiencing hypnosis, *not* with the tests the person must pass for us to decide that he can experience it. In other words, I am concerned with the question, "What can I do to help this person experience hypnosis?", not with the doubt, "Is this person able to use hypnosis?" I ask myself, "What do I have to do, what do I have to change in *my* thinking, actions, and attitude, in order to help this person use hypnosis?" For I know that if the person is of average intelligence and emotional stability and has the right mental set, hypnotizability is not a concern at all. The right mental set, as explained elsewhere by the acronym TEAM (Araoz, 1982a) and based mainly on T. X. Barber's (1969) research, is a combination of *trust* in the clinician, in the ability of one's mind, and in the hypnotic procedure; of reasonable *expectations* about hypnosis; of an *attitude* of cooperation and desire to try something new for one's own benefit; and, finally, of true *motivation* to improve, grow, or change for the better.

If a client does not respond to hypnosis, *the method* of approaching the person is changed. The client is not dismissed as nonsusceptible to hypnosis. The clinician asks himself what has been neglected and/or ignored in the existential encounter with the person and literally starts again or gives himself another chance to reach the person. More will be said about this later when discussing induction.

Hypnotizability as a concept reflects a way of understanding what hypnosis is all about. My approach views hypnosis as a natural process of using one's mind, which is indeed different from the ordinary way of thinking—an *alternate* mentation, but natural and normal nevertheless.

In sum, there are several concepts related to hypnotizability. First, hypnosis is now often understood as the activation of the right cerebral hemisphere (e.g., Erickson and Rossi, 1981; Watzlawick, 1982). The new discoveries of our "two brains" provide a sound physiological base for the generally accepted explanation of primary and secondary process thinking, derived from psychoanalytical theory. Fromm's (1977) detailed description of ego states in hypnosis may be translated into bilateral hemispheric terms. Her "observing ego," for instance, is obviously a function of the left hemisphere, while her "experiencing ego" fits neatly into the right-hemispheric functions.

Second, based on the research on imagination and brain bilaterality mentioned above, the New Hypnosis considers all normal persons (of average intelligence, health, emotional and social development) able to use hypnosis. If there is no hypnosis, it is not because of the client's low hypnotizability score. Disregarding the value of such scores, the clinician needs to consider his awareness of the client's thinking mode and emotional needs.

Third, hypnotizability thus turns into *hypnotizing ability*, the flexibility of the therapist to adapt to the client's current thinking mode. This belief derives from Erickson's constant awareness of the current and changing inner experiences of the client (Erickson and Rossi, 1979, 1981; Erickson, Rossi, and Rossi, 1976). Some clients may require *training* to obtain the mind skills needed to experience hypnosis, which becomes the fourth concept related to the old hypnotizability concept. There are no "non-hypnotizables" in the general population. Therefore, the clinician feels a special responsibility to tune into the client's unique psychological makeup.

Hypnotic Depth

Disregarding far from accurate scores of hypnotic depth (Tart, 1979), the New Hypnosis is concerned with increased *imaginative involvement*. In this sense, effective imagery activity *is* hypnosis, the right hemisphere being "the image-making brain" as described by Oyle (1976), who deals specifically with physical disease from a Jungian perspective. The more involved the person is in his inner reality (imagery in the broader, etymological sense of the word) the more intense his hypnotic experience and the less active his generalized reality orientation.

Self-hypnosis

Consistent with the learning approach, the New Hypnosis emphasizes self-hypnotic practice. From the very first, clients are encouraged to engage in this type of mind exercise, and for this purpose cassette tapes are often made specifically for each client's use at home. These cassette tapes are mere training aids—like training wheels when a child is learning to ride a bicycle—soon to be discarded when the person has acquired the skill of self-hypnosis.

It has become commonplace to state that all hypnosis is self-hypnosis. This was the contribution of the Nancy school, as Baudouin (1922) explained at great length. An interesting study conducted by Fromm and her associates (1981) compared the differences between hetero-hypnosis and self-hypnosis. In some cases, it seems, the hypnotherapist becomes a distraction for the hypnotic experience. The study found, for instance, that imagery is richer in self-hypnosis but that age regression and hypnotic hallucinations were helped by the presence of the hypnotherapist. It is easy to understand that most people would be afraid of engaging in the two latter hypnotic experiences alone. The presence of a trusted hypnotherapist acts as a protection against unexpected events which may take place while age regressing or hallucinating.

Others, like Sacerdote (1981), believe that only spontaneous hypnosis is self-hypnosis, since there is always a "teacher" (book, audiotape, or previous experience with a hypnotist) in any self-hypnotic experience. He further claims that deep hetero-hypnosis is a prerequisite for a meaningful self-hypnotic experience, though his evidence is far from convincing.

The New Hypnosis, following the teachings on heterosuggestion made popular by Coué and Baudouin, links hypnosis with daydreaming (both sharing similar mental dynamics) and describes hypnosis as a goal-directed daydream. Diamond's (1983b) cognitive skill model of hypnosis stresses the choice of the individual before starting the hypnotic experience. This is the "goal" set for the hypnotic experience. What does the person want hypnosis for? Let us assume that the goal is to overcome psychogenic depression. Imaginative involvement or daydream material will then be utilized to counteract depressive cognitions, such as self-talk, imagery, selective choice of negative feelings and bodily sensations.

Therefore, the insistence on self-hypnosis fits into the general framework which theorizes hypnosis as a *natural* mental activity. Self-hypnosis is the means by which people are taught to use the natural process of self-talk, cognitions, and imagery for their own benefit, not against themselves.

In the traditional approach, the hypnotist is paramount, whereas the New Hypnosis places more responsibility on the client—the real locus of control—and perceives the hypnotherapist as a guide or teacher who helps the person develop the natural skill of engaging in hypnosis.

APPLICATION OF HYPNOSIS

In this section I shall review the techniques used by the New Hypnosis, the way the understanding of hypnosis is applied in the clinical setting. This leads us to discuss two main topics; induction and utilization.

Induction

From a perusal of the traditional literature on hypnosis, it would seem that induction is perceived as a first, discrete step in the hypnosis process (see *Syllabus of Hypnosis*, published by the American Society of Clinical Hypnosis in 1973 and still used in its training seminars). It is as if induction had some value in and of itself: Induction produces the state of hypnosis; induction leads to trance.

On the other hand, the New Hypnosis prefers naturalistic and indirect methods of "switching" from ordinary mental activity to hypnosis—from left- to right-hemispheric functioning. In so doing, induction becomes part of a continuum with the hypnotherapy itself; induction is a moment of centering oneself or of focusing (Gendlin, 1978) on one's inner reality in order to eventually bring it to conscious awareness in most cases. In practice there is little distinction made between hypnotic induction and hypnotherapy. The focus is less on technique and more on awareness of the client's here-and-now reality. Consequently, what follows must be understood according to that basic principle: Induction is already hypnotherapy. The therapist does not have to arbitrarily find something for the person to pay attention to, as in a traditional induction; rather, a simple invitation to become aware of one's body may be all that is needed to effect that passage from reality orientation to inner orientation.

The effective induction is based on close observation of the client (as will be explained further in Chapter 4): her breathing; the movements of her eyes, hands, and shoulders; the general position of her body; facial expressions; and so on. These behaviors are observed not to interpret them, either to the client or even to oneself, but to help the client become more aware of herself. A typical induction might go something like this:

> Notice the weight of your hands on your lap. . . . What else do your hands notice? Check it now . . . a feeling of warmth, perhaps. A slight breeze in the air. The temperature in the room. . . . If you would separate your hands now you may notice other interesting sensations, such as one feeling lighter than the other. Which one is it?

In any instance the therapist has many choices for the induction since attentive observation always yields more items than those with which one can possibly work at once. In the above example, I focused on the client's hands. But at the same time, she is breathing and her breathing rhythm could have been used.

She is also resting her feet somewhere—another possible focus of attention for induction. One may list such natural possibilities and many more. The main point here is that *induction proceeds from the client* so that she can become more aware of her inner self. By becoming aware of one's current experience, one is led slowly into one's inner realities. Self-awareness leads to the subconscious.

The general principle to remember is that any spontaneous behavior of the individual can be used effectively for making the switch from ordinary thinking to hypnotic thinking. Thus, we may select from gestures and ask the person to repeat them in an exaggerated way, allowing anything that comes to mind to build up in her. Then we lead her to become aware of any feelings engendered by this brief experience. Let's assume the person is saying, "I can't go on like this anymore," while at the same time making a fist with her right hand. The therapist may then ask the person to repeat that gesture a few times while making the same statement. If the arm was shaking when the fist was made, this should also be repeated. Usually three or four repetitions elicit something new. In the current case, the person may say that she is getting angry or that she remembers now, as coming from nowhere, an incident from childhood. The therapist then proceeds with the new material.

If, on the other hand, nothing is elicited after repeating the gesture a few times, the therapist should continue, remembering that at any given moment the client is offering more behaviors than it is possible to use therapeutically.

Besides gestures and bodily feelings (which I call somatics, in general), the therapist must pay close attention to statements and to the language used, rather than merely to the content of it. The above example of the person saying, "I can't go on like this anymore," could be used as an instance of an important statement. We recognize important statements by their affect content, the current context, or information we have obtained previously from and about the client.

The point of all this is that these elements, provided by the client without her full awareness, offer the most effective and most natural vehicle for hypnosis. The practitioner of the New

Hypnosis observes the person carefully and respectfully, utilizing any of the elements provided by the client herself. I have grouped all these various elements into three categories, namely, *somatics* (gestures, facial expressions, shifts in body position and awareness of body parts or functions), *language style* (whether the person uses one representational system or inner sense more frequently than others), and *important statements* made by the client while with the clinician (see further in Chapter 4).

Any one of these elements can be employed to switch the person's mental activity from reality orientation to inner orientation. And this effort is the preferred form of naturalistic induction of the New Hypnosis. It should be added that when clients, for whatever reason, request more traditional inductions (even with the use of a disc or a pendulum), the respectful flexibility of the New Hypnosis practitioner will probably allow use of these methods as well.

In order to make the preceding discussion more practical, I shall return now to the language used by the client and describe how a nontraditional induction proceeds. The clinician trains himself to become a keen observer of the client's current preferred thinking mode—whether with a predominance of mental pictures, sounds, smells, tastes, or somatic sensations—as is revealed in the client's language. Language, among other things, reflects one's thinking mode at the moment in the choice of figures of speech, adjectives, verbs, and speech forms. The clinician becomes aware of these pieces of information and waits for the client to use them. Then the client is invited to get more involved in the mental representations which are reflected in her speech. Let's assume that the client is talking about a general feeling of despondency, unhappiness, and boredom with life in general. The following might be instances of the language style used: "My whole life stinks"; "I find myself in a hole"; "I'm in the dark"; "I've lost my taste for everything"; or "Nothing sounds right to me any more." When a client is encouraged to mentally experience what her speech reflects about her thinking mode, the hypnotic goal is reached, namely, connection with subconscious processes.

From this point on it is suggested to the client that she use to the fullest the mental images that spontaneously develop. Let's follow this imaginary example. In any of the above instances the client will not be invited to talk more about it, but be urged instead to utilize whatever experience lies dormant behind the subconscious choice of figures of speech. The client may be told:

> Just stay for a moment with that mental image: "My whole life stinks." Feel the stink in your nostrils. How does that smell affect your whole body? Get into it as fully as you can. Feel enveloped by the stink of your life. "My whole life stinks"—keep repeating this until you feel it in your whole being.

Notice that logical, rational "translations" of the figures of speech are not encouraged, as other forms of therapy might do by asking clients to elucidate the figures of speech and inviting them to explain what they mean.

In this sense the clinical use of hypnosis emphasizes a thorough and relaxed involvement in one's inner awareness, with the messages coming through not from the external world or the conscious mind. These messages—each of which raises a consciousness of self—are more than intellectual insights. They are true *insights*, a new way of viewing oneself and one's world. The ancients, with a more religious attitude than we have, talked about inspiration, as if a god blew into one's mind some precious message. The techiques described in Chapter 3 explain several different ways to establish a connection with the inner mind, either through spontaneous imagery or through somatic manifestations.

The task of the hypnotherapist is to help clients become familiar with this mode of relating to themselves, which our Western upbringing and education generally do not develop or encourage, and to produce the conditions favorable for a full involvement in their inner reality. This double task of the hypnotherapist is accomplished experientially and thus simultaneously.

Because of the gradual progression of inner, imaginative involvement, I prefer to refer to hypnotic height (Araoz, 1982a) rather than depth. Perhaps my preference comes not only from the fact that "high gear," "high expectations," "high spirits," and other such expressions all have very positive connotations, but also from a clinical incident that happened many years ago. Following the traditional language of hypnotists, I was working with a young man and saying, "You can get even deeper into your present experience—deeper now than when you started," and so forth. Later he told me that he did not want to embarrass me while he was in hypnosis but that depth meant danger to him. Images of being buried deeper had come to his mind. Besides, anything "in depth" meant something that needed deep concentration, that was difficult and thus something that made him tense, anxious, and uneasy. On the other hand, to say that "you are getting into a higher level of inner awareness" may frighten someone who is not comfortable with heights. The clinician will have to be careful about the use of words and expressions. The moral of the anecdote is that the hypnosis experience can be perceived either as deep or high, depending on the client and the circumstances.

In sum, whether the person has reached some arbitrary level of hypnotic depth is not as clinically important as the constant concern of the clinician to have clients as totally involved in their inner mind experience as they are able to be.

Other methods of naturalistic, unobtrusive "induction" are the following:

(a) Becoming fully aware of one's body sensations and then focusing on one (e.g., breathing) until subconscious material emerges;
(b) Repeating a significant statement (e.g., "I can't take it anymore") until inner subconscious processes emerge into consciousness (see Chapter 4);
(c) Reliving in one's mind a past experience, as opposed to merely talking about it;
(d) Becoming aware of one's body energy (called "aura" by some) until the health forces activating the parasympathetic nervous system are felt;

(e) Focusing one's mind on a positive, constructive, possible goal in one's future, thus rehearsing it in one's mind;
(f) Simply allowing the person to be silent, while suggesting that the subconscious can start to work at that moment of "doing nothing" without the awareness of the conscious mind (Erickson and Rossi, 1981).

This short list is a mere sample of possible nonritualistic inductions. They are all in line with my experiential description of hypnosis as a "letting oneself go into a goal-directed daydream to the extent that one dissociates oneself from one's surrounding reality and becomes engrossed in one's inner reality" (Araoz, 1982a). These methods of induction lead to an *alternate* state of awareness without "altering" one's mental functioning.

Induction, then, becomes a natural "invitation" to connect with one's inner, subconscious self. It is always personalized, tailored to the client with whom one is dealing. It is not ritualized, following a definite sequence of steps as in Traditional Hypnosis. In the latter case, this ritual may include arbitrarily asking clients to look up as if focusing on the inside of their skull or to lift their arm to shoulder height and then slowly allow it to drop or "reversely levitate" (do we reversely stand when we sit?), or to do some other maneuver similar to these. The ritualized induction becomes sacramental for many traditional hypnotherapists. In the Catholic teaching a sacrament is a ritual (such as baptism) which ex opere operato (by its own action) produces a particular effect. In that case, God's bestowing a specific grace. In Traditional Hypnosis, some people take the induction rituals as if they, by their own power, had some intrinsic value. Magic and hypnosis are still connected in the popular mind, probably encouraged by these attitudes which mechanize what should be a highly individualized, personalized communication between client and therapist.

The New Hypnosis, then, seldom thinks of induction as a discrete and separate step, after which the client is ready for the therapeutic work. Induction is already part of hypnotherapy, and frequently the goal for which hypnosis is used is mentioned from the very first moments of the hypnotic induction.

Utilization

In Traditional Hypnosis there is often a definite attempt at re-programming clients' minds by excessive use of direct sugges-tions. It is curious that Neurolinguistic Programming professes loyalty to Erickson's teachings, yet he disliked the cybernetic model applied to humans: "Programming is a very confusing way to tell a patient to use his own abilities" (Erickson and Rossi, 1981, p. 217). Instead, "you try to accept the patient's ideas, no matter what they are, and then you can try to utilize them" (p. 13). He was obviously referring not just to conscious ideas but also to any mentations coming from the patient's subconscious mind.

Utilization, therefore, is not programming. It is, rather, the ef-fective use of the hypnotic experience for the benefit of the client. It responds to the question, "How can hypnosis be used most effectively with this individual?" The techniques employed in the New Hypnosis are justified only as methods for utilization, as every clinical example in this book shows.

In this area lies the very significant difference in the use of hyp-nosis by the trained and experienced therapist (using either Tra-ditional or New Hypnosis) and by the hypnotist—whether in the entertainment field, an investigation, or in a setting of mere be-havior change such as smoking cessation—who follows a method to "hypnotize" a person leading to a specific goal. In the latter case, there is no acceptance of whatever ideas may come from the subconscious mind (to paraphrase Erickson's earlier quote) and, consequently, there is no utilization of them. To put it an-other way, the lay hypnotist does not want to be distracted from the specific goal of hypnosis by uninvited subconscious material. The hypnotherapist's goal, on the other hand, is less concrete and more open-ended; she works mostly with the subconscious material emerging during the hypnosis experience, moving ap-propriately from the first to the second or third level of therapeutic intervention (first level centers on the symptom; second level on immediate connections; third level on psychodynamics and historical material).

On the other hand, the hypnotist stays at the first level, disregarding new subconscious material. I witnessed an example of this at a night club show where the hypnotist was getting volunteers to sing like famous performers. Shortly after starting to sing like Elvis Presley, a woman became upset and began to cry. The hypnotist distracted her from whatever subconscious element was triggering her emotional reaction and quickly stated: "At the count of three you won't be upset anymore. You'll feel fine. One—very fine and very happy. Two—feeling very good. Three— you feel terrific, ready to sing like Elvis Presley." Instant therapy! Instant repression, yes, and no utilization at all.

CONCLUSION

This chapter has dealt with the specialized issue which touches the very core of the experience of hypnosis. This is the issue of human change. In the light of this complicated concept I have discussed hypnotizability, hypnotic depth, and self-hypnosis as essential ideas for the clinician's understanding of hypnosis. I have also discussed induction and depth, as well as utilization, as techniques to apply to the understanding of hypnosis.

Techniques for
Inner Transformation

The ultimate goal of any hypnotic intervention in therapy is change. But since change, to be effective, must come from one's inner self, I prefer the ancient Greek expression, *metanoia*, associated with early Christian conversion. For a conversion to be genuine, the person had to accept the new belief and way of life "from within." Anything less did not count. Metanoia means, then, a drastic change in one's perception of oneself and one's world. It is a change in one's *world image*, the constant element at the root of all human emotional problems. The world image, as explained by existentialists, is the mental image we have formed of our world. This often does not correspond exactly to what the real world is. This discrepancy leads us frequently to want to conform the world to our world image. As long as this is impossible, we suffer emotional stress and pain. The solution to this conflict is a change in our world image, which slowly has to become more in harmony with the external world, as long as we assume that the latter cannot be changed. Thus, it can be said (Watzlawick, 1978) that all people plagued by emotional problems suf-

This chapter is adapted from an article published in *Medical Hypnoanalysis*, July, 1983 (Vol. 4, No. 3).

fer from their world image. In a sense, then, this becomes a meta-diagnosis, underlying all other specific diagnoses.

To achieve this metanoia or special transformation there are several major techniques used by the New Hypnosis. This chapter will describe them and give practical applications. These techniques fall into several categories as the chart shows. For brevity's sake and to avoid repetition, 12 techniques will be discussed (see Table 1), though many more could be listed. However, upon close consideration, all other techniques fall under one of the 12.

LEVELS OF INTERVENTION

It should be remembered that all psychotherapy must proceed in an orderly fashion. Kaplan's (1976) suggestion for sex therapy applies as well to any form of psychotherapy oriented to change. There are three levels of intervention which cannot be altered without risking confusion and waste of time. The first level aims at *the symptom* in itself. Many of the techniques described in this chapter are effective at this level, though the second group (mind techniques) are mainly geared to the next two levels. In my ex-

Table 1
New Hypnosis Techniques

	Somatic Techniques	
	Relaxation	
	Somatic Bridge	
	Subjective Biofeedback	
	Mind Techniques	
Dissociative	*Time Alteration*	*Paralogical*
Dissociation	Transfer of Inner	Paradox
Activation of Personality	Resources	Parable
Parts	Emotional Bridge	
Materialization	Reliving	
	Mental Rehearsal	

perience, more than 80% of all therapy cases can be resolved at this level.

If the clinical intervention directed at the symptom does not yield change in the person's life, the clinician moves on to the level of *insight I*, at which the person is helped to recognize surface connections with the symptom. For instance, a day of depression may be preceded by a visit from a disliked relative. From 12%–15% of those who do not respond at the first level can be helped by insight I. Only when these two levels of therapeutic intervention do not produce results does the therapist move on to the third level—*insight II*—at which psychodynamics connected with one's personal history are dealt with.

The psychoanalytical bias is to ignore or bypass the first two levels, often prolonging the therapeutic intervention needlessly. The evidence accumulated from the beginnings of behavior therapy (see Stuart, 1970, on iatrogenic disturbances) indicates, first, that symptom substitution is far from universal and, second, that to ignore the first two levels of intervention often precludes growthful change in the individual client.

SOMATIC TECHNIQUES

These are techniques centered on the bodily experience. In *relaxation*, for instance, frequently the simple and constant act of breathing becomes a focus of attention, leading to a change of self-experience. In *somatic bridge*, a slight pain or discomfort in any part of one's body is the beginning of greater awareness and integration, a bridge to the subconscious mind. In *subjective biofeedback* one uses one's body to monitor emotional reactions.

Relaxation

All hypnotherapists know the value of relaxation. Relaxation gives the parasympathetic nervous system a chance to take over. Tension or lack of relaxation occurs when the sympathetic nervous system is active longer than is necessary to take action or to face a threat or danger. What this technique of relaxation attempts to achieve is activation of the parasympathetic nervous system, that mechanism which brings all our bodily systems to optimal functioning. In practice, I find that as long as the client does not have any breathing difficulties, it is helpful to start with his normal breathing. The approach may be very simple. For instance, I may say something like this:

> You are breathing now. Please pay attention to the way your body *likes* to breathe. Don't force anything. Don't stop anything. Just *breathe* and find out what is your body's *rhythm* of breathing—its breathing tempo. Let is happen. Plenty of time. No rush. Just breathe. While you breathe, think of relaxation . . . as if you were watching your whole body, your *whole* body, relax—really r-e-l-a-x. Enjoy the relaxation. Let it happen. Right now.

The relaxation chatter continues as long as the person needs it to become relaxed. It is always useful to encourage clients to close their eyes when they blink naturally. I find myself speaking in the following terms: ''You just blinked. Next time it happens, notice how restful it is to blink. Perhaps you may even want to put your blinking *in slow motion*, while your whole body *enjoys* this experience of relaxation. All systems *slow down* while you enjoy the experience.''

For those who have some breathing difficulty (such as asthma, emphysema, hyperventilation, or similar conditions) and consequently may have associated breathing with discomfort, the technique of relaxation must start elsewhere. In this case, the therapist may use any of the traditional hypnotic techniques (eye fixation, arm levitation, different kinds of visualization, etc.) or ask clients to remember a situation in which they felt very relaxed. Once the situation is decided upon, more and more details are introduced in order to ''re-produce'' the same somatic experience of relaxation the person experienced in the situation currently remembered. Let's assume the client identifies as a relaxing scene one night during a ski trip when he could not sleep and sat by a dying fire, while the snow was falling outside and everybody else in his party was deeply asleep. The therapist can then build on this scene until the person reexperiences the peace and relaxation of the original situation. (The 25 "images" suggested by Kroger and Fezler [1976] are very helpful to build on the relaxing scene offered by the client.)

As a back-up technique in those cases where a person is too tense or distracted to follow instructions to relax, the paradoxical approach of muscle tensing and relaxing in fairly rapid succession is beneficial. It demonstrates dramatically to the client the sensation of relaxation. Once this is accomplished, one may proceed to the other methods described earlier.

Relaxation is a general technique since practically every person we deal with can benefit from it. However, the main point is not so much muscle relaxation as *inner peace*. This is important to remember because a person who is worried, guilty, or anxious with negative thoughts cannot obtain the type of relaxation we are dealing with. In practice this means that the hypnotherapist must address himself to the client's inner reality. It can be done in conjunction with the instructions suggested in the previous paragraphs. For instance:

> While letting your breathing *blow away* your tensions—like tiny particles of dust leaving your tense muscles—let your breathing *fill* your mind with *good* thoughts. Let your breathing fill you with *peace* and inner *serenity*. Breathing in comfort. Breathing in good feelings—peace, quiet, tranquil thoughts. Distractions will come and go. Let them just fly through you. Your inner *peace is* the important thing right now.

Somatic Bridge

The general concept of this technique is taken from Watkins' (1971) affect bridge. Rather than being used to activate older ego states by focusing on a feeling common to something both current and past, the somatic bridge is similar to the Oriental "taitoku" or body-thinking. As such, it is a way of utilizing awareness of one's body to facilitate awareness of repressed feelings, since authentic self-transformation (metanoia) must include the whole being rather than be merely intellectual. Because of this, the somatic bridge is effective with people who are too left hemispheric, or who have never developed intuitive, symbolic, and emotional capacities, which are the functions of the right cerebral hemisphere.

The technique is introduced when clients feel "they have nothing to talk about," or feel "flat," with no emotion. The hypnotherapist invites the person to simply sit there and pay attention to the body: "The goal here is not to talk about it but to *experience*. What parts of your body are you aware of now?" the clinician may ask. "Just *become aware* of one part. Stay with the awareness. Don't talk. Don't do anything. Let distractions come and go. Just enter the awareness of your body more fully." Only after clients have become involved in body awareness do they describe what was being experienced. Then, the hypnotherapist may continue: "Now, let the awareness of your body *lead you* to something which is hidden in the recesses of your mind. Just wonder what will come up: memories, images, joys, pains. Whatever comes is OK. Your inner mind will speak to you in a new way through your body. Take your time. Let it happen and you'll *learn* important things about yourself. *You'll be* surprised and pleased."

Many mental health workers agree that clients must get in touch with their feelings. The problem often becomes how to accomplish this. The somatic bridge is a surprisingly quick and effective technique to facilitate this. Frequently a host of meaningful memories and psychological connections rush to awareness, giving the client significant therapeutic material to work on.

This technique is rich in therapeutic potential. Often when the client concentrates on one part of his body, mental images occur. These, then, should be followed, as in the case of the man who started to be aware of his left foot, describing it as "more like a slight itch on my big toe." I invited him to concentrate on that itch, "to get more into it." At that point the man frowned and said, "Like a current going up to my groin." I suggested that he visualize the current: its force, thickness, and speed. He saw it as a line of a silvery color, perhaps even made of silver, and added, "But I don't know what it means." Typical of most people in our culture is the impatience *to know* and the discomfort with mere experiencing and being. I replied, "You will know soon enough. Now, just *stay* with that silvery line. *Feel* it going from your right toe to your groin. Does it end there? What happens there? Take your time and stay with the silvery line." This sensitive respect for any material coming from the subconscious mind is not a form of anti-intellectualism but rather a holistic approach to being alive. Understanding follows experiencing. The silvery line didn't end there. It soon became a powerful light that enveloped his whole body. I encouraged him to enjoy the new energy with which he was in touch. He connected it with "the energy that keeps me alive, the force of life in me, life itself." After this experience he talked about his mental attitude in the last few days which had been rather negative and pessimistic. He had been ready "to fold his tent," as he put it. This experience made him think more positively about his future, about enjoying life more, about giving himself more time to play, have fun, and relax.

This example is typical.The meaning discovered through this approach seems to emerge without the laborious left hemispheric activity of analyzing, evaluating, and "thinking." And what makes this therapy always interesting and full of surprises is that the hypnotherapist does not have to wonder where to go next, what to do next. She simply follows carefully and respectfully what the client's inner mind offers naturally, spontaneously and, at times, even playfully.

The somatic bridge may be used any time a client expresses a somatic awareness. Whether it is tiredness, a slight pain, a headache, or anything similar, it becomes surprisingly therapeutic to stay with it, to allow it to become the focus of attention, and then to let it develop, paying attention to mental images, memories, and psychological connections.

It should be remembered that a careful diagnosis is always assumed. Psychotics should not be exposed to this technique carelessly, since it may lead to a frightening—and dangerous—dissociation, with a sense of lack of control. The experienced hypnotherapist will assess the ego strength of individual clients before introducing them to this or any of the somatic techniques.

Subjective Biofeedback

This technique starts with a mental image, or a memory, provided by the client. Then attention is paid to the way the body reacts to that mental activity. Finally, meaning emerges out of this connection. Let's test it first with ourselves. Imagine a very sad experience; visualize it in detail. Then attend to your body's reaction to it. Just notice it and become aware of the fact that there is harmony between mind and body. The Cartesian separation between the two is more didactic than real, as Oriental philosophy and medicine teach us. Do the same again but this time think of something very exciting and joyful. Stay with it and relive as many details as possible. Next notice how your body—some part of your body—is reacting to the joyful and exciting experience. At the end, check if any meaning emerges from this spontaneous connection. If not, repeat the exercise until your conscious mind becomes aware of this link and understands in a uniquely subjective manner what this connection means to you.

It is important to experience subjective biofeedback first in ourselves before we try it as a technique with clients because, generally speaking, most Westerners are very unfamiliar with these experiences. We tend to concentrate too much on thinking (left hemisphere) at the expense of inner experience and feeling (right hemisphere). A remarkable exception to the rule is the experience of mystics who have frequently been labeled anti-intellectual. One of them stated it succinctly: "What satisfies the soul is not to know much but to taste and savor things internally." He was Ignatius of Loyola, the founder of the Jesuits, one of the most intellectual and highly educated groups in the Catholic church.

After having tasted and savored this subjective experience internally, we may think of applying it in our clinical work to help clients "get in touch with their feelings." Ikemi and Ikemi (1983) refer to the inability to express feelings as *alexithymia* and have

coined the term *alexisomia* for the condition that makes it difficult for a person to express how his or her body feels. Subjective biofeedback helps overcome these conditions. This technique
may be used with important statements (e.g., "I really love this
woman") or non-planned gestures (e.g., a spontaneous fist, or
both hands going to one's chest). The client is asked to close his
eyes and to repeat the statement (to himself or out loud) or the
gesture several times, while checking what happens in his body.
Whatever emerges from the inner mind becomes, then, the next
focus of attention for continuing the therapeutic work. The following example illustrates use of somatic techniques.

A Clinical Case

A.D., age 24, had been referred to me for psychogenic impotence, which had precluded him from copulation since his first
attempt at age 17. I asked him to concentrate on his impotence
and to become aware of his bodily reactions to it. He first did not
experience anything in particular. I helped him become more relaxed and to focus on a pleasant scene, a vacation place where
he could feel carefree and comfortable, without anything to do,
but with the freedom to do anything he wanted. While he was
there, in his favorite mountain place, enjoying the majesty of the
Canadian Rockies, I asked him to shift his attention to his sexual problem. Immediately he noticed a sharp tension in the back
of his head. I invited him to stay with that sharp tension and to
allow any mental image that might accompany it. He responded that it felt like an ice pick but, surprisingly, caused no pain,
but a clear, sharp tension. I suggested that he concentrate on the
sharpness of his experience.

He felt at this point that the ice pick became very long and
reached all the way to his chest. Now he experienced a tension
that started in his head and went to his chest. "Do you visualize
the connection between your head and your chest?", I asked.
After a few moments of silence, he said, "It's like a wave that
goes back and forth—a dark wave, heavy, and wearing me out."
My answer was: "Even though it may be uncomfortable, stay

with it for a while; experience it fully." A few moments passed and he said very slowly and quietly: "My head, my heart, my penis—they are all connected." I continued to encourage him to utilize fully every new spontaneous item coming from his subconscious mind: "Experience this connection fully. What is the connection? What does it feel like? Take your time to feel it. You don't have to understand it. You don't have to talk now. Just experience." After a few moments of intense concentration on his part, I added: "Say to yourself that your inner mind has found a connection between your head, your heart, and your penis. Trust your inner mind. In the next few days you will understand more about this connection. Welcome anything that your inner mind wants to do with this connection. You *know* you can enjoy sex; your heart *wants* to enjoy sex fully. Will your penis cooperate now or later? That'll be your great and pleasant surprise. Let's leave it to your inner self to put the three together."

This was the end of the first session. At the next session, a week later, he reported that the problem was still there but that, somehow, he felt confident and he knew it was going to be all right. He had been with his current female friend three times— two of them sexually. But even though "nothing happened" he had felt more relaxed and hopeful. Hypnosis was used as in the first session, adding the imagery of a relaxed sexual experience without mentioning copulation.

The third week, A.D. had been sick and had seen his lady friend only once. However, during the four days that he had been in bed, he had practiced his relaxation and self-hypnosis, giving himself the message that his inner mind was in the process of working on his problem and soon he would have a pleasant surprise regarding it. In the session, he concentrated hypnotically on a positive sexual encounter with his female friend.

At the fourth session, A.D. was exuberant. He reported successful intercourse twice. I invited him to stay with his good feelings and to focus on them next time he saw his female friend. The goal, he had to remember, was not performance but enjoyment without worry. He spent about 15 minutes in hypnosis rehearsing a relaxed sexual encounter where he and his friend were absorbed in the enjoyment of being together.

The fifth session, 10 days later, was a celebration of success. He had enjoyed intercourse three times and was looking forward to the next opportunity for intimacy with his woman friend.

I saw A.D. twice more, one week later and, again, one month thereafter. His new behavior was being maintained and he was feeling more confident with each successful copulation. Three months later he called me on the telephone to report continuous success. Six months after that call, he and his friend came to see me because they were contemplating living together but had some practical questions. At this time, both referred to his "old sexual problem" as something from the remote past, an almost forgotten difficulty of long ago.

One may speculate on what dynamics were at work in effecting this change in such a short time, when the therapeutic intervention remained at the first level of the symptom without going on to the second or third levels mentioned earlier in this chapter. It may have been a case of subconscious, healthy integration of his beliefs—now corrected through his awareness of a unifying energy in his whole being (head, heart, and body)—and his sexual expression. He came from a background of strict sexual abstinence outside of marriage but in experiencing a unification of his total being he also experienced himself as the person he was at the time, not as the child who had received the injunction of sexual abstinence before marriage. This may have freed his inner mind to allow his body to react in a mature way to the current situation with his female friend.

As in some of the cases reported by Erickson (e.g., 1935), the client experienced growthful change without understanding the dynamics responsible for it. By using this approach the clinician has many humbling opportunities like this. He is obviously helpful to the client but without knowing how his intervention elicited the desired outcome. Effective therapy does not depend on the clinician's understanding of the process leading to such beneficial change, as Watzlawick (1976), Rossi (Erickson and Rossi, 1979), and others have reminded us.

Traditional hypnotherapists are familiar with ideomotor techniques. These consist of procedures to elicit involuntary movements of the fingers as an indication of "thinking" which is going on below the level of the client's awareness. Ideomotor responses are effective in bringing subconscious "thinking" to the conscious level. "It is believed they come from unconscious sources," explains Edelstien (1981), "and clinical experience tends to support this belief" (p. 53). Earlier in the same chapter he had stated that "it is difficult, if not impossible, to offer clear explanations of how or why (these techniques) work. They do work, however, and there is no need to deny patients the benefits of their efficacy until the theorists have evolved suitable explanations" (p. 47).

Traditional hypnosis elicits these ideomotor responses in a planned, almost contrived manner. Even though the New Hypnosis does not reject these technqiues in appropriate clinical situations with clients who may benefit from them, it prefers more naturalistic approaches. The somatic bridge and subjective biofeedback are such naturalistic techniques. They, too, are ideomotor manifestations of subconscious "thinking." Rather than artificially concentrate on the client's fingers, the therapist proceeds as indicated in the previous sections. The "awareness" that comes from bodily sensations has the same source of subconscious thinking as the traditional ideomotor techniques. The somatic bridge and subjective biofeedback can be used for the same purpose as traditional ideomotor techniques, namely, to uncover subconscious thinking and to deal with material which was "protected" (defended) from awareness.

In sum, the somatic bridge and subjective feedback techniques are ideomotor, though less artificial and more natural and spontaneous than the traditional finger responses.

MIND TECHNIQUES

Although all of the 12 techniques we are discussing are essentially "mental," i.e., involving one's mental capacities, the next group does not focus primarily on the bodily experience as the somatic techniques do. Mind techniques are more specifically used to alter our perception of our problems and to facilitate metanoia, the difficult transformation which starts at our world image and translates itself at the behavioral and relational levels.

Dissociative Techniques

Dissociation. Let's start with an example. A woman is very angry, sad, and frustrated because her three grown children have "abandoned" her after her three-year separation from her husband of 36 years. She has tried to talk to them, to explain, to confront them, but all to no avail. They promise they'll call and keep in touch but long weeks go by without any sign from them. When she finally calls, they either respond with surprise at her complaint or tell her clearly there is nothing to talk about and that's the reason they have not contacted her. She had been in therapy discussing this for six months. No progress was noticed either in her children's behavior or in her depressed mood, though she had become more involved in outside activities with different groups of mature adults.

Many years could be spent analyzing this woman's reaction to the children's "abandonment." An alternative (emergency) procedure is to use dissociation. She is asked to have a pleasant or funny daydream. The daydream is in order to leave the emotional pain behind, "so that you don't have to be with the pain all day long." This is a method she can learn in order to stop the emotional pain, at least for a while. In the office she is kept in her pleasant daydream for several minutes at a time. She is made aware of how different (even good) she feels while she is daydreaming. She is asked to practice this exercise every day. Later, this technique is coupled with mental rehearsal (which will be explained later).

In many cases where the therapist feels frustrated and helpless with a client, dissociation is a first step to lead a client to further growth. In the case of the woman just mentioned, her "little journey of the mind," as she started to call it, gave her relief several times a day. Later she started rehearsing mentally new things she would do, other people she could start to count on; and in less than two months *she* had decided that her children were emotionally toxic to her and that she would not contact them unless they did. This was a sad decision, indeed, but by that time, she had prepared herself for her "new life" at the ripe age of 66.

Activation of personality parts. This technique, like the somatic bridge, is also taken from Watkins (1978) but modified in the sense that the emphasis is less psychoanalytical. It could be called *healthy personality split.* It consists of making a habit of *not* considering any feeling, thought, mood, or action as "emanating from me" but as "coming from a part of me." Every time clients say, "I feel . . . ," or "I keep thinking . . . ," the hypnotherapist reminds them to check what an opposite part in them is thinking, feeling, or saying. Clients are asked to continue doing this in private. "Check the parts in you" becomes the constant injunction. If the person is depressed, for instance, one may ask to listen to what the depressed part is saying inside. Then, "Is there another little part, perhaps, that is not agreeing with the depressed part? Let's hear what that part is saying." This is a way of enlarging one's awareness by realizing in practice that seldom is one's whole being involved in any inner experience. By such examination of the whole picture of one's existence, a person can realize that "at least a tiny part of me is not in total agreement with the depressed (angry, frustrated, etc.) part."

What the hypnotherapist does is to allow clients to really identify with the new part, to become the new part completely, and to be aware of how the new part feels. Rather than just *talk* as the new part, it is imperative to help clients experientially to *become* that part. Then, and only after this experience, it may be useful to discuss what the part may mean, why it triggered the memories it did, etc. Rather than ask clients to describe the part to me, I suggest that they take their time to experience deeply that new part. Later, we talk.

This technique has many possibilities, limited only by the hypnotherapist's and the client's imaginations and willingness to "sound silly."

Materialization. This is another form of dissociation in that it separates clients from their problem. However, the difference is essential. Here the problem is not left behind but visualized and experienced differently. Let's suppose a man starts the session by stating he is confused. (Notice that traditional therapy would probably encourage the person to talk more about it, to explain the confusion.) Using the New Hypnosis, the therapist would encourage something experiential (right hemispheric), suggesting that the client imagine his confusion in some material form or object familiar to him. Can the confusion become a fog or a deep darkness or a cacophonous sound or like the experience of falling from a great height? Is there any mental image for the confusion? The client is asked to close his eyes, to relax (using the techniques explained earlier in this chapter), and then to concentrate on some mental image that the thought of his confusion might trigger. Usually, and if the hypnotherapist gives the client options for visual, kinetic, auditory, and even olfactory and gustatory mental images or representations, the client gets in touch with some symbol of his psychological state. If not, memories arise or other associations are readily made.

This is an appropriate place to note that techniques are always a means to an end. If one does not work, another one can be used for the same purpose.

The general idea is to check whether the problem appears symbolically. If clients are able to produce a mental image or symbol, the therapist asks them to stay with it and concentrate on the feelings and inner experiences in order to make them completely their own. At this point, an expansion of consciousness or awareness takes place. Even though we are discussing techniques individually and separately, the expert hypnotherapist will be quick to mix and combine different techniques in order to attain the desired effect which, to repeat, is a change in one's perception or world image so as to be able to react differently to the situation or issue which produces the problem or symptoms.

Time Alteration Techniques

These are interventions which use time distortion in one way or another. Three of them refer to the past and one to the future. Even though the New Hypnosis, because of its experiential nature, deals mostly with the present, it is simply naive to attempt to avoid references to the past or the future. As humans, we are both trapped by time and free because of time. Time alteration techniques utilize our temporal reality experientially, not to analyze the lessons of the past or the dreams for the future, not to make sense of them and understand them, but to experience fully the inner reality of things past or projected into the future in order to own completely that aspect of our being.

Transfer of inner resources. When clients feel helpless or discouraged by current situations, many interventions can be used if the therapeutic purpose is to alter that affect so that they feel more positive about themselves. The transfer technique has several variations but essentially it consists of focusing on past situations in which the person acted extraordinarily well and felt unusually good. This situation is used hypnotically, reliving it in great detail, eliciting as much of the positive affect as possible, and repeating the experience several times if needed. Then, the person is asked to check—again, experientially—whether any of the inner resources used in that positive situation might have some value in the current situation that makes the person feel helpless, discouraged or, in general, negative. As in all these techniques, allowance must be made for slowness of movement. Frequent injunctions are: "There is no rush." "Take your time." "Try to stay with that question." "Check whether any of the personality traits you used then could be helpful now." (An example of the application of this technique appears in Chapter 8.)

Another way of applying the transfer technique is to start with the negative situation and the affect it elicits, then go to a positive situation of the past with all the good feelings it engenders, and finally return to the negative scene with some of the resources which, used in the past, made the person feel good and positive.

Case Example

An example may help, showing how techniques can be combined in clinical work. This case uses transfer, as well as subjective biofeedback and mental rehearsal. A 39-year-old woman, divorced for the last five years, had just broken up with a man with whom she had been very involved for the last four months. She wanted to make the relationship more serious and he didn't. She decided to stop seeing him, but later became very unhappy, lonely, and anxious to meet "the ideal man." At the therapy session after the breakup, I employed a transfer technique.

Cl: As I told you over the phone, I still feel miserable, though I know I had to break with him. And I also feel proud that I did.

DLA: Check now if you experience the sadness some place in your body. Take your time to become aware of your body, breathing, sitting there. Your eyes closed, trying to feel some peace.

Cl: (after about 90 seconds) I'm becoming my sadness. It's painful (starting to cry silently).

DLA: Stay with the sadness and pain just for a few more moments. You are the sadness, the pain.

Cl: (Quiet, but with the beginning of a frown. Concentrating but breathing in a relaxed manner.)

DLA: Now, when you are satisfied that you have experienced your pain and sadness, change the mental picture to something completely different. Think now of another situation in your past that was very good for you, that made you feel terrific, happy, in control, competent, proud of yourself. Let that memory fill your mental screen. Take your time and let it happen. Your inner mind will choose a very positive scene for you to relive now.

Cl: (Silence for about two minutes of relaxed breathing and general body relaxation. Then a bit of a smile, slowly becoming a full smile.)

DLA: Whenever you're ready, you may want to tell me what scene is coming up. Don't rush. Stay with it and absorb it completely. You are there, you feel terrific.

Cl: (after about four minutes) My new apartment. No husband. He's gone forever. My own place, finally. I made it!

(This woman had been in a very violent marriage. Her husband had beaten her and threatened the life of Nicole, their two-year-old girl. She had left him in the middle of the night, moved in with her parents who protected her until she found her own apartment. Her husband, in the meantime, had been taken to jail for embezzling from a large corporation, where he was an officer.)

Th: Stay with this picture and all these good feelings. You are safe, you're free. You are proud of yourself. You saved yourself and your child. Now this is your place—all yours to share with Nicole whom you have saved. (After about five minutes of encouraging her to fully relive all the good feelings she had experienced then, I continued.) Now go back to the sad scene, to your present pain and sadness. But take with you some of the good feelings you had when you were first in your apartment. Use some of those good things in your current sadness and pain.

Cl: (after a few moments) Yes, it feels good. I'm doing it. This sadness is OK. It will pass. I'll be OK.

The session continued along the same lines. Mental rehearsal (to be explained later in this chapter) was added at the end so she could experience herself beyond the current sadness.

Emotional bridge. Although this intervention is also taken from Watkins (1971) who calls it the *affect bridge*, to avoid calling it "the modified affect bridge" or some other such name, I have labeled it *emotional bridge*. The reason is that this technique is less psychoanalytical than Watkins'. When a client is experiencing a particular emotion and the therapist has indications that it may be related to past experiences or events, the emotional bridge is a very helpful intervention. Let's assume the client, a woman, is feeling a general confusion, whose origin cannot be understood in terms of current events in her life. At this point, I may suggest that she stay with the confusion; that she concentrate on physically (bodily) experiencing the confusion to the utmost; that she let any memories and mental images connected in any way with confusion emerge slowly or quickly: "Your whole being is now confusion." This often is enough to establish a psychological link between the present confusion and significant past events where confusion was also experienced.

If there is no immediate reaction, I become more explicit and say something like this: "You have been confused before. Perhaps not exactly like now. Allow your inner mind to connect this confusion with some other confusion of the past. Take your time, relax, and just let confusion—here and in the past—absorb all your being."

In this way, the current emotion acts as a bridge to other past instances of the same feeling, allowing the person to broaden her awareness and thus to learn something new about herself. This learning about oneself, frequently mentioned by Erickson while working with his clients, is the main purpose of the emotional bridge. The connection with a previous similar emotional experience leads to either separating the two or learning how to handle the current situation from the way the previous one was handled.

Reliving. Somehow regression has obtained a negative connotation for many therapists and clients. However, regression in the service of the ego (Kris, 1952) is by no means a new technique in psychotherapy. I prefer to refer to it as *reliving* previous experiences. Others have described this intervention in detail (see Weitzenhoffer, 1957; Wolberg, 1964). I want to stress that this technique is essential when a person seems to be fixated on some traumatic event of the past. By reliving it, under the guidance of the hypnotherapist, the client obtains a new control over the event. This approach, combined with *activation of personality parts* (described earlier) works well with people who have experienced emotional deprivation in childhood. For example, the technique became an important part of the therapy with a woman whose mother kept her in a small closet between the ages of four and six while she went about the house chores. The woman relived the event, but at that point she also saw herself as she was now, a grown-up woman who knew how to deal with little children.

She was able to console the young self, providing it with all the support, understanding, and protection it needed. This woman learned to implement this technique every time she felt depressed, since she had realized her depression was linked to those cruel scenes of her past.

Mental rehearsal. In our Western world, we have been taught to think logically, to test reality, to be objective—all functions of the left hemisphere. Mental rehearsal bypasses logic and moves ahead in time. It operates in the future, as opposed to the other time alteration techniques which move back into the past. Mental rehearsal is the imaginative effort to experience oneself in the future, the way one believes one can be: "Now, jump ahead and experience in your imagination the self you are, without the problem you have. The problem is gone, resolved, finished. You are now without this problem. *Like* yourself, *enjoy* being without the problem. You are OK now. How does it feel? Check the way your body reacts to this new reality of being."

Athletes are being taught to mentally rehearse as much as they practice in vivo. Businessmen and -women are encouraged to fantasize successful situations and to experience in their minds the feelings they elicit (Araoz, 1984b). Actors are taught to become the character they portray by using their imagination to do it. Many methods of therapy employ psychovisualization, "in the mind's eye" technique, and "movies of the mind." In other words, mental rehearsal has become a valued method of facilitating change in many diverse situations.

It should be remembered that often, when people "worry" about a forthcoming event, what they are doing is mentally rehearsing *against themselves.* They use the same mental mechanism, but negatively. And in most cases, it works! It keeps up the negative feelings and "prepares" the person to fail or suffer in the upcoming situation. Mental rehearsal utilizes the same process for one's benefit and fulfillment. Every time clients in therapy talk about accomplishing something, about changing in some way or other, I suggest that they "see" themselves changed.

The centuries-old Virgilian statement, "They change their being because *they see themselves* changing," is a brief definition of mental rehearsal.

Paralogical Techniques

These are interventions which attempt to communicate directly with the right hemisphere of the brain. Watzlawick (1978) has discussed masterfully the language of the subconscious mind, and the reader is encouraged to become acquainted with his work. Paradox and parables have been used by many of the great masters in both Oriental and Western civilizations, though most psychotherapy training has ignored these ancient teachings and the style proven effective through many centuries.

Paradox. The point of the paradox is to use an indirect method where a direct one would encounter resistance. The work by Weeks and L'Abate (1982) should be read carefully in order to understand clearly the value and uses of paradoxical interventions. Within the New Hypnosis approach, paradox is made experiential. The woman whose daughter was looking for reasons to commit her to a mental hospital, said one day that "she was falling to pieces, she was in a real hole." I suggested that she see herself, in her mind's eye, becoming crazy, falling apart at the seams. We spent some time with this exercise and at the end she said very firmly: "I won't give her (the daughter) the satisfaction of seeing me crazy. I'm not crazy. I'm very upset but I can manage it."

Another client, considering leaving his wife because he was so much in love with another woman who was pressuring him to move in with her, was told to see himself with the other woman; to go over in detail the circumstances of living with her, keeping house, buying groceries, cooking meals, etc. After this exercise, he realized that he was not ready to make the decision to leave his wife, that he did not want to take the next step (moving in with the other woman) at this point.

These two examples may serve to remind us that paradox as

understood in the New Hypnosis—to menally live something which is considered incredible but possible—helps a person confront the whole truth about the dilemma and, by so doing, make a decision rather than remain between the two horns of the issue.

It is possible to consider any symptom as a symbol of subconscious dynamics. The presenting problem, though real in itself, has roots in the inner mind. This concept does not mean that the clinician should bypass or ignore the symptom. Assuming the symptom *is* a symbol, right-hemispheric focusing through hypnotic techniques will be more effective than mere talk, since symbolism is the purview of the right hemisphere.

Paradox treats the symptom as a symbol so that it yields its meaning. In the above-mentioned case of the woman whose daughter wanted to hospitalize her, the anxiety was in part a symbol of her fear of displeasing and ultimately losing her daughter. When the client used her imagination not to avoid the thought of becoming crazy but to experience herself insane, she realized she did not want to go along with her daughter and, in so doing, she tapped previously ignored inner resources. One of the comments made when she was processing her change in attitude was that losing her daughter's affection was very sad but preferable to being crazy.

The man, who in hypnosis imagined concretely what it would be like to live with the other woman, understood that his feeling greatly in love was a symbol of his need for excitement and that it would weaken when the current thrill was gone. He came to the conclusion that he wanted to take his marriage seriously and to put all his energy into making it exciting.

This clinical manner of proceeding has several advantages. It reaches the subconscious dynamics quickly but it does not require a detailed understanding of them, as we saw earlier in the case of the man with sexual impotence. However, by reaching the subconscious, this approach often does produce a new connection between the inner and conscious mind, bringing the unknown dynamics to awareness. But this awareness usually happens *after* the experience in hypnosis: Understanding follows experience. Because of this new awareness the individual is able

to make new decisions, thus producing growthful change, as the
two above examples show.

Parable. Some authors call it metaphor (e.g., Gordon, 1978),
but parable is the word that indicates the technique of presenting a short story conveying a message (moral) unique to the person addressed, though not explicit. The hypnotherapist must be
very sensitive to clients' needs before using this very delicate tool,
since the parable is always a subtle form of interpretation of what
clients are experiencing in order to present to them some material
which will "connect" with that state of mind. The parable can
be personal, as Erickson showed often ("When I was a youngster,
there was a horse . . . "), or poetic ("The woods, asleep through
the winter, burst into life when spring called"); but in either case,
the goal is to bypass consciousness—resistance, evaluation, analysis, intellectualization. Watzlawick (1978) has called this technique
a "dream in reverse," citing as an example the woman who complained of "frigidity," to whom Erickson told the story of de-
frosting her refrigerator. What could have been a story dreamt
by that woman, the therapist presented as a means of reaching
the subconscious level of mind activity.

The more cultured the hypnotherapist, the richer his reper-
toire of possible parables. Those stories that have survived the
centuries hold eternal truths which can be used effectively in therapy, rather than the inane stories some therapists create on the
spur of the moment attempting to utter profound wisdom.

I also find that the parable can be used symbolically. For instance, in case of impotence, arm levitation becomes a very meaningful analogy of how the inner mind can influence the conduct
of one's body.

CONCLUSION

Techniques are always means to an end. Consequently, no
technique is justified (ever!) unless the hypnotherapist knows
what the current situation of the client is and what effects can

be expected from that operation, intervention, or technique. No technique has value in itself. Because of this, the experienced hypnotherapist usually mixes techniques in his clinical practice.

The novice should avoid the temptation to "collect" techniques the way a cook collects recipes. A therapeutic technique is always *a response* to a given situation; it is part of the interaction taking place between two human beings—in the unique situation of therapy—one of whom is the hypnotherapist and the other the client. But, regardless of the situational role, the human interaction between these two people must remain the most important aspect of this special relationship. The response given by the hypnotherapist to what the client needs or is experiencing at the time takes the form of a technique. If any therapeutic technique is not a response, it is at best useless and at worst damaging to the relationship between client and hypnotherapist. Thus the therapist should be extremely respectful of the client. Rather than saying "I now want you to do this or that," (why should another human being do anything because *you* want it?), the therapist will be more effective with a more permissive approach. It could be expressed in terms of "inviting," "suggesting," or "proposing." For instance: "You may now want to try. . . . " "I might suggest that you try. . . . " "May I propose that you do this or that?"

Resistance is often a healthy reaction of the client to the intrusive manner of the therapist. If the therapist's approach is changed, such resistance often disappears altogether.

As mentioned before, the techniques described here are used by the New Hypnosis. The truth is that traditional hypnosis employs them as well. The main differences between the two approaches should be outlined once more (Araoz, 1982; 1983). First, the New Hypnosis assumes that hypnosis, being a natural mental function, is within reach of every normal person with the motivation to learn this way of "thinking" or using one's mind, called hypnosis. The second difference, a corollary of the first, is that hypnosis is considered a skill, not a trait, which can be learned with proper guidance by anyone wanting to learn it. The therapist, then, is mainly a teacher or facilitator and the locus of control is the client, not the therapist. Consequently, the notion of hypnotizability is disregarded. Clients are not tested for the ability to be hypnotized, but the therapist is ready to try diverse approaches to help the person into the mental activity, primarily right-hemispheric in nature, designated as hypnosis. The onus rests on the therapist's ability and flexibility to help the client use hypnosis, not on the client's ability to be hypnotized, which is always assumed.

The third difference is that the process of induction into hypnosis is not ritualized but "naturalistic," starting with the reality of the client's inner experience of the moment. The fourth difference is that the depth of hypnosis is of much less concern than in the traditional approach. Finally, the understanding of what hypnosis is all about is independent of the classic psychoanalytic background prevalent in traditional hypnosis.

The techniques described fit within this context. There is no intention "to own" these techniques nor to imply that they were developed by the New Hypnosis advocates. They simply lend themselves to comfortable use by those who do not follow the traditional approach to hypnosis.

Part II

Characteristics

This part of the book highlights two main characteristics of the New Hypnosis approach: client-centeredness and personal experience. The model for therapeutic work, following a sequence of steps to reach the inner experience of the client, is also outlined.

Although client-centeredness and personal experience are the main trademarks of the New Hypnosis, these two characteristics comprise many others, as will be detailed in the following chapters. Most of the qualities that make hypnosis work depend on the attitude of the clinician, rather than on the mechanical application of certain techniques, as we all know. However, for those unfamiliar with hypnosis, it is necessary to stress this last point since many still believe hypnosis has some type of magical value.

4

Client-centeredness

This chapter focuses on an essential characteristic of the
New Hypnosis, one which places it firmly among experiential
therapies, as well as among those of the humanistic/existential
clinical mode. This characteristic is a complete centeredness on
the client, going beyond what Rogers and his followers have accomplished (see Barrett-Lennard, 1959; Boy and Pine, 1982; Halkides, 1958; Hart and Tomlison, 1970; Meador and Rogers, 1979;
Rogers, 1959, 1961; Rogers et al., 1967; Truax and Carkhuff, 1967).

First I shall present a clinical case in order to illustrate this client-centeredness and then I shall outline in detail the process of
hypnotherapy which utilizes New Hypnosis principles and methods, as summarized in the OLD C paradigm.

A CLINICAL CASE

Referred by her internist, Mrs. L had been experiencing dizzy
spells, never fainting but very afraid that she would do so. Mrs.
L was 46 years of age, married 25 years, with two boys away in
college at Ivy League universities. Her husband was president
of a bank, and both were very involved in their church and many
community organizations. Mrs. L spoke in a cultured, refined
way, with a slight British accent, though she had never lived in
the United Kingdom.

After the preliminaries of the first session, I asked her to tell

me about her dizzy spells. (The verbatim transactions which follow are numbered in order to make it easier to refer to them later
in the chapter.)

Mrs. L: They are just dreadful. Bloody dreadful and annoying,
   I'd say. (#1)
DLA: What happens in your body when you *start* to feel dizzy?
   (#1)
Mrs. L: That's a quaint question. Let me see . . . what happens
   in my body? You mean, inside of me? (#2)
DLA: Yes, but I mean physically, in the body. (#2)
Mrs. L: I guess I just feel dizzy (silence). (#3)
DLA: Start *before* you feel dizzy. Put it in slow motion. Close your
   eyes and go over the sequence now, very slowly. (#3)
Mrs. L: (not closing eyes) Slow motion . . . I guess I'm going
   about my own affairs. (She is looking at me and I gesture to
   slow down while smiling at her.) Then, I suppose, I start slowing down and feel rather weak and become dizzy. (She said
   this in a different tone of voice, almost slurring her words.) (#4)
DLA: Check how you feel right now. What's happening right
   now inside of you? (#4)
Mrs. L: I guess . . . (#5)
DLA: No. Don't speak now. Just check how you are feeling and
   go with the feeling or with any sensations. . . . Check what
   you are aware of now. (#5)
Mrs. L: I'm afraid I'll faint. I feel dizzy. (#6)
DLA: You *can* faint here. This is a good place to faint. Perhaps
   you'd want to . . . let yourself . . . faint now. (#6)
Mrs. L: (in a plain, non-British tone) No, I couldn't do that. (re-
   suming her British accent) I shan't do it! (#7)
DLA: Stay with that statement for a while. Repeat to yourself,
   "I shan't do it!" Modify the statement any way it feels good.
   "I won't do it!" "I shan't do it!" . . . Maybe you do have the
   power to avoid fainting. Repeat to youself that you won't do
   it. (#7)

Mrs. L was quiet for more than a minute while I repeated "I
shan't do it" or "I won't faint" gently but forcefully every 10

to 15 seconds. She was visibly relaxing her guarded and controlled attitude, and had finally closed her eyes for the last half minute or so. After that time, she opened her eyes, smiled, and said:

Mrs. L: Dr. Brown said you are a hypnotist. Are you hypnotizing me? Is this hypnosis? (#8)

DLA: I'll tell you sort of a secret. I really don't believe in hypnosis in that sense. And no, I'm *not* a hypnotist. I have no power over your mind. I can't make you do what you don't want to do. It's always self-hypnosis. *You* were getting in touch with some of your inner resources you had forgotten you had. I was just leading you to do it. What happened when you kept repeating to yourself that you wouldn't faint? (#8)

Mrs. L: (relaxed, in a quiet voice and without the British accent) It feels good. The whole business of fainting is part of the sham. (returning to her controlled self) I know this is ridiculous. Just because I state I shan't faint, it wouldn't happen, would it? I would still faint. (#9)

DLA: Part of you feels, thinks, "It's ridiculous." But another part feels good about it. Both parts are you and I'd like to take both parts of you seriously. (#9)

Mrs. L: I don't understand what you might mean by that. (#10)

DLA: Just what you stated. On the one hand (one part in your personality) you feel good saying to yourself that you don't have to faint. On the other hand (a different part of your personality) you feel ridiculous that you have control over your fainting. Am I correct? (#10)

Mrs. L: Yes, I suppose so. But you talk about this as if there were two discrete personalities in me. I can't accept that. (#11)

DLA: You are absolutely right. You should *not* think of two different personalities but rather of two *aspects* of your personality, like, for instance, the way you act towards your children and the way you act towards strangers. It's you in both cases but using different aspects of your personality. Does that make sense? (#11)

Mrs. L: I suppose so. Yes, it does. So, what would you like me to do right now? (#12)

DLA: Close your eyes again. Say to yourself, "I have control over

my fainting,'' and check how this statement makes you react.
Fine. Yes. Close your eyes, like that, and gently say to yourself, "I have control over my fainting." (#12)

Mrs. L: (barely audible now) I have control over my fainting. (#13)

DLA: Keep relaxing while you're breathing, while repeating the
same statement. (pause) Very well. Just like that. Check now
how your body is reacting to your statement. Is there any part
of you which seems to disagree with your statement? (At this
point Mrs. L's breathing became almost forced, as if gasping
for air.) (#13)

Mrs. L: (making a fist, pointing to her chest and without her British accent) I feel the tension right here. (#14)

DLA: Please, stay with that tension. Go with it. Check what happens. "I have control over my fainting." Keep your eyes closed
to avoid distractions. Check the tension in your chest while
you keep your fist pointing to your chest. Keep your fist, yes,
like that. (#14)

Mrs. L: (still in her non-British voice) I *know* what the trouble is.
Yes, a part of me and a part of me. But I can't do it. I can't
say it (emphasizing with her fist). (#15)

DLA: It's OK. Don't do it. Relax for a moment. Breathing nicely. Now focus on what you *know* is the trouble. Let your inner mind reflect on it. (She is becoming more relaxed.) Check
that tension in your chest. (She smiles to indicate that that is
not a problem now.) Go back to the parts in your personality. (tension in her face, frowning) (#15)

Mrs. L: (in her non-British voice) Yeah, there are two parts, all
right. (long silence) (#16)

DLA: Imagine an animated cartoon in which those parts of you
are represented . . . as if you were watching a cartoon on television. Your two parts appear in the cartoon. Do you see them?
(She smiles, nodding yes.) Let the cartoon roll, watch what
you see in your mind's eye. Hear the two characters speak.
Are you with it? (She nods yes.) When you are ready, you may
repeat what the two parts in you are saying, if you want me
to know it. Just what you see and hear in the cartoon you are
mentally watching. Are you still watching? (She says "Yeah"

in a very low voice). You may want to tell me what the two parts are saying. (#16)

Mrs. L: (in standard American English, with angry feeling) One is saying, "Your whole life is a farce. You are a fraud, a *lie*! You can't stand your husband and his phoney ways. You know he's chickenshit. And you hate the damn churchgoers, too. His *friends*. They're all chickenshit, hypocrites, like you." (silence, heavy breathing, and tears) (#17)

DLA: How does this part look in your mind's eye? (#17)

Mrs. L: (silence) It's me . . . when I was . . . I guess before I was married. (#18)

DLA: OK. Listen to that part once more and check now more carefully how your body is reacting to all this. (#18)

Mrs. L: (silence) I'm fine now. . . . There was tension before, but now I'm fine. It's the truth, isn't it? My life is a sham. I'm admitting it now. (smiling) I can't believe it. I can't believe what I said. But I don't regret it. Maybe I'll leave the whole lie behind. You know, I *will* leave the lies behind. I hate them . . . I can't believe what I'm saying. But I mean it. I'm not sorry. Not at all. (silence) (#19)

DLA: What about the other part? Is she still there? Can you hear what *she* is saying? (#19)

Mrs. L: Oh, yes. (with an angry smile) She wants me to ignore my true being. "You're OK. You have what you always wanted: money, status, power, security," she yells. I hate her phoney British accent. I do have all that but I've paid for it with my own being, with my soul. I'm a prostitute of sorts. . . . She's old, ugly, and phoney. Her soul is wrinkled. (silence) (#20)

DLA: Allow both parts to calm down a bit. Perhaps they can talk to each other, interact. . . . Both parts belong to you. (#20)

Mrs. L: (slowly and in a relaxed voice) I don't want that. I want to get rid of the phoney me. I'll fire her. I want to be true to myself. (laughing) I don't have to faint now. All that dizziness was my way of avoiding the truth, the lies in my life. I don't want to faint now. . . . I'll be happy. I know what I have to do. (as if thinking out loud) I have to see the lawyer and walk away from my phoney life once and for all. I'm still young enough to live true to myself. (silence) (#21)

DLA: How does your body react to your decision to stop the lies and change your life? (#21)

Mrs. L: (silence) Great, really great. I feel relieved. I feel good, very good. (opening her eyes) I knew it all along but I was unable to face it. I'm relaxed now. . . . (#22)

DLA: Just as an assurance, go back to the two parts and let your true self fire the phoney self. Want to do it now? (#22)

Mrs. L: (closing eyes) I might as well do it. (#23)

DLA: But this time see the true self as grown up and mature, the way you are now. (#23)

Mrs. L: No, I like her young. (silence) I know I'm not young anymore but I like to be young inside. (silence) Yes, my true self takes over. My phoney self is gone. (silence) It feels so good. . . . (#24)

DLA: Stay with this good feeling. Keep your eyes closed and absorb the good feeling. Let any mental image come to you. Let any sensation come . . . let any memory come . . . while you feel good. . . . What comes to mind? (#24)

Mrs. L: (silence) My phoney self is gone. I haven't loved my husband in many years. It feels good to admit it. A nice picture comes to mind . . . I'm overlooking mountains and valleys on a beautiful fall day. I'm at peace. I'm free! I'm happy. I'm alone. No Warren (her husband) anymore. . . . Everything in my life is good . . . no anger anymore. Just peace. (#25)

DLA: Go with these feelings. Take in the beauty of the place, the colors, the cool air. Listen to the nature sounds. Feel the comfort of being there . . . young inside . . . ready to enjoy life to the full . . . in truth . . . in peace. . . . (#25)

Mrs. L: Yeah. I like this. (silence while she keeps a relaxed smile) (#26)

DLA: This is your place of peace and truth. You may want to come back to it many times in the next few days and feel good again. (#26)

Mrs. L: Yeah, I'm happy and I know now what I'll have to do. (#27)

DLA: I guess we'll give your true self a whole week to do what
she has to do. (#27)

With this the session came to an end, though we spent a few
more minutes discussing her experience. Her British accent did
not come back; her whole attitude was more relaxed and friendly
than at the beginning of the session. Mrs. L, who now asked me
to call her "just plain Mary," stayed in hypnotherapy for the next
three months on a once-a-week basis. During the following seven
months, until her divorce was settled, she saw me once every
three or four weeks.

Before I explain the OLD C model, using the preceding session as an example of it, I think it might be helpful for the reader to quickly review the same session once more in order to notice the times in which Mrs. L (from now on to be called Mary
at her request) presents nonconscious material (either figures of
speech, significant statements or somatics) which I use to lead
her further into her own inner reality or experience of the here
and now.

THE PROCESS OF HYPNOTHERAPY

The above transcript of a typical hypnotherapy session illustrates the client-centeredness of the New Hypnosis at the experiential (right-hemispheric) level of mental functioning. Without
formal induction or rituals that are connected in most people's
minds with hypnosis, Mary experienced a meaningful "transformation." She was not encouraged to verbalize but to experience.
She was asked to go with whatever was coming up from her inner mind. In this session there was little discussion as such; no
analysis of reasons or pros and cons; no values clarification. In
other words, my intent throughout the session was to bring Mary
back to right-hemispheric activities whenever she reverted to logical, reality-oriented thinking, as in transactions #5, #8, and #9,
among others. Mary, exemplifying all patients, was gently but
firmly directed to focus on her inner realities as they became man-

ifest in the interaction with me. She was invited *to experience* anything that spontaneously came up, not *to talk* about her problem. The therapy session becomes then an emotive laboratory where the client experiences herself in a new way, thus learning new aspects of herself. Emphasis is on *the process* of the interaction which manifests internal realities, not on the content of what the person says (though the latter is obviously not ignored).

The sequence as followed with Mary is what I consider the basic paradigm of the New Hypnosis. In outline form it may be represented by the OLD C acronym: O for *observe*; L for *lead*; D for *discuss*; and C for *check*. These four steps can be described briefly as follows:

1. *Observe* reminds us to pay close attention to what the client is offering nonconsciously in the therapy session. To facilitate this observation, three main areas are considered:
   • Language style
   • Significant statements
   • Somatics (any changes in the body of which the person can become aware, such as internal sensations and external movements)
2. *Lead* the client to experience more fully any of the above manifestations of internal realities. This is the core of the process, avoiding explanations, interpretations, analysis, or intellectual insights. Focus is on right-hemispheric activity.
3. *Discuss* the experience of Step 2 above only *after* it is completed, not while it is happening. The therapist must allow the client to *fully* experience her internal reality and only then process it intellectually.
4. *Check* the genuineness of the above process by going over Step 2 and monitoring how the body reacts to the process. This check will either confirm and validate what just took place or necessitate further work.

As illustrated in the clinical case presented above, this client-centered process can be started without preliminaries and does not take long to complete; one session is more than adequate to proceed from the beginning to the end of the process. In this way it has similarities with Gendlin's (1978) focusing and tends to generalize because of its naturalness and simplicity, teaching clients to use it for their own benefit outside of the therapy sessions. Obviously the four steps of this sequence overlap, as the previous transcript shows. The OLD C model is heuristic and it serves to explain the hypnotherapy process from a New Hypnosis perspective.

Observe and Lead

The therapist's most important concern is twofold: 1) to be in touch with the client's inner experiences during the time both persons are face to face; and 2) to pay close attention to the three areas of observation so that the client can be led to inner experiences. Most therapists have been trained to attend to past experiences (even if the past is limited to the previous few days) and to the content of the client's verbalizations. The OLD C model, in part, tries to avoid those two pitfalls which make much psychotherapy useless and ineffective. This paradigm helps to accomplish what many therapists consider one of their aims, namely to make it possible for clients to be in touch with their feelings. By paying attention to the nonconscious processes manifested during the therapy session in the language style, the significant statements, and the somatics, the therapist can really *lead* the client, that is, help her to become aware of her feelings and to react in accordance with the new control of these feelings obtained through the OLD C process.

Language style. The first area to observe is *language style*, not what the language expresses (its content). By this I mean the choice of words, figures of speech, sensory modality, analogies, and so on. At some inner level people choose the expressions they use in language, though this choice is far from consistent as the study by Coe and Sharcoff (1983) indicated. Our "inner senses," with which we construct mental images (inner representations of external realities perceived by our five sensory receptors), control the choice of elements in our language style. Expressions may be kinetic, such as "I can't stand it any longer," "It doesn't sit well with me," or "It makes me sick." *Visual* expressions are quite common in our culture: "You see what I mean?" "Let me throw some light on the subject." "I'm in the dark." "It sounds great," "It's music to my ears," and "Listen to your body" are *auditory* expressions. These three types are the most common in Western culture, though it's not rare to find manifestations of *taste* and *smell* in our daily language. Thus, "He came out smelling like a rose," "She stinks," "I smell something fishy here," "It was a delicious evening," "My mouth is watering," and "I have a sour taste about this" are examples of the two nondominant senses.

I must stress the need for the hypnotherapist to observe the language style of the client. When the person uses an expression that seems to reflect an inner sense, the therapist will do well to invite the client "to stay with it, to experience what it feels like to (have something sound great, or see something clearly, or feel stuck and the like)." If the client does not respond right away and tells you that she can't get into it, don't insist; wait for the next opportunity in either language style or significant statements or somatics.

Another aspect of the language style is that of the mental images reflected in words. Every one of these can be used therapeutically within the OLD C model. Let's assume the client says he feels "light as a kite." Rather than ask him to expound on it left-hemispherically by explaining what he means, what happened, since when is he feeling this way, I invite him to employ this image right-hemispherically, I ask him to let himself feel light as a kite, to really *get into* it with all the details that may emerge from his inner mind, to allow himself to go with this image as far as it will take him. However, if nothing comes up, I do not insist but, rather, wait for the next figure of speech or pictorial sentence to try the same approach until he can capture meaning through greater awareness of his inner mind's processes and messages.

In the case of Mary, mentioned above, there were no obvious examples of language style. Towards the end (#24), when she said "It feels so good," I encouraged her to go with the image evoked by this feeling. This invitation transferred her to a beautiful outdoor setting on a mild fall day (#25), which she will use as her place of peace and truth whenever she needs it.

Significant statements. The second area of careful observation on the part of the hypnotherapist concerns the important phrases or statements made by the client in the course of the session. The clinician must judge which statements are significant from the specific context in which they are uttered and from the affect accompanying them, as well as from the matter at hand being focused on.

The case of Mary presents several significant statements, starting with #7 when she said ''I shan't do it.'' This statement was not elaborated on logically or analytically. It was used then and once more (#8) to help her become aware of her true feelings. Later (#12 and #13) the same statement was enlarged and modified. This led Mary to the issue of control over her own life, as the session progressed, and to her decision to stop the elements of dishonesty and falsehood in it. Had I used the initial statement in a left-hemispheric way, *discussing* with her issues of control, it probably would have taken much longer to reach the point she reached in that first session. The experiential method connected with her subconscious awareness about her life and tapped her inner strengths to do what she had to do, in spite of her reluctance shown in #15. Congruent with my desire to facilitate ''right-hemispheric'' work, I discouraged her from forcing herself to break the resistance by sheer willpower, but led her further into her inner experience. I also used the animated cartoon technique (#16) by which she would feel safer giving voice to that ''part'' of her which existed underneath the sophisticated, British, and overly controlled exterior.

Somatics. The third general area to observe in order to lead the client to a fuller experience of herself is that of body sensations as well as gestures, posture, and facial expressions. To embrace them all, I use the word somatics. By calling a client's attention to body sensations, as I did with Mary in #1, #4, #5, #14, and finally

#18, the clinician allows other important inner awareness to take place. Because of #4 and #5, Mary used a significant statement (#7) which, in turn, led her to be aware of the control over her life. In #14, the concentration on her chest tension made it easier for her to break through the resistance against facing the phoneyness of her life. Lastly, her concentration on her body in #18 confirmed for her the direction her life had to take from then on (#19 and especially #21 in which Mary "interpreted" the meaning of her dizzy spells and fear of fainting).

Subconscious material that proves important to the client is often triggered by asking a client to repeat a gesture or to exaggerate it. When Mary made a fist spontaneously in #14, I encouraged her to use that unpremeditated gesture which helped her come face to face with her fear of doing what she knew she had to do, namely, step out of her dishonest lifestyle.

In subsequent sessions Mary used somatics in similar ways, allowing a sensation or spontaneous gesture to lead her to a new awareness of herself. If one theorizes that somatics are manifestations of the inner mind, it makes sense to take them seriously and *lead* them so they can develop and reveal the meaning they might have for the individual client.

Thus, guided by careful observation of the client's language style, significant statements and somatics, the therapist is able to *lead* the client to discover the meaning of whatever the latter's subconscious may bring up through the process of enhancing that experience. The therapist does not interpret, analyze, or connect the experience with previous material. This discipline of *leading* comprises the whole range of therapeutic interventions.

Let's assume a client mentions how he drives himself, working at three jobs, having hardly any time to spend with his family or relax. To arbitrarily select one interpretation (he's trying to prove something, probably that he is the best or that he can be what his father thought he'd never be) has the danger of stopping the subconscious flow. First, the client will probably start focusing on the question and talk about what he "is trying to prove," regardless of the direction in which he might have been going before the therapist's question. Most clients, at some level, are trying to please the therapist. Second, feelings associated to what the client is talking about are stifled, because they are aborted rather than encouraged. These feelings are real for the client at the moment but are not allowed to emerge. In the above example, the client may feel elated, excited and free, driving himself as he was describing. But he may also feel guilty, anxious, and depressed. All these feelings may be far from evident to the client or the therapist. By asking an interpretative question, the feelings are abandoned and a new intellectual search is encouraged, distracting the client from the true inner experience of the moment.

Leading also must be done with sensitivity to the changes in mood experienced by the client. The prevalent mood or affect should be utilized. In the transcript, Mary mentioned that "the whole business of fainting is part of the sham" (see #9) but quickly returned to her controlled self after that. To have used this to lead her would probably have been premature (as #15 shows) and, consequently, it would have wasted time. Only later (#17) when she focused on it again was the time right to lead her, as her resolution in #19 indicates.

Discuss and Check

After the client has had a chance to get in touch with her inner experience, she should process it intellectually. In the OLD C model, this is the place for *discussion* as such. Because the main activity during the hypnotherapy session is not conversation, as the case of Mary showed, it is useful for the clinician at the beginning of the session to refer to occupations other than "talking." One may suggest that therapist and client *work* or *focus on* something. The discussion is incidental to the experiencing and only in order to integrate it with the understanding of the same. In the illustrative session above, very little part of it is devoted to discussion, e.g., #8, which points to the fact that often discussion is not needed. The client, all by herself, may have reached the intellectual understanding needed for the mental integration of the inner experience.

The last step in the OLD C model is referred to as *check*. This check is also part of the integration process. It consists of reverting to the current experiencing once the client has accepted something intellectually. This experiencing may take the form of physical sensations (#22) or mental imagery (#25). Indeed, both usually are present. This gives the therapist and the client assurance that the whole self of the client is assimilating or has assimilated the previous experience resulting from the *lead* step. Often I may ask the client to check if any part inside of her seems to disagree with what has happened. If the result of this quest is peace, comfort, and/or positive imagery, the process is completed.

If, on the other hand, the final check produces tension, either physical or mental, that tension (a form of somatics) is used to lead the client once more, reverting to Step 2 of the OLD C model and proceeding from there.

CONCLUSION

To conclude, then, the approach outlined in the previous pages is most thoroughly client-centered. The totality of the client's experience in the here and now is used to make change possible. Verbalization is in the service of inner experience; it is not the main means to work hypnotherapeutically. Rather than using verbal free association, the New Hypnosis works with free association of inner experiences, either mentally (mainly through imagery) or physically (through body sensations). These free associations are facilitated by the therapist's *leading*, as explained above.

The New Hypnosis uses "the inherent capacity of the organism to develop all its capacities in ways which serve to maintain or embrace the organism," to quote Rogers (1959). This approach is successful when the therapist's own mental images are allowed to do their healing and therapeutic work without interference from understanding and reason. To echo the play *Man of La Mancha*, too much reason might be the worse type of folly. Or, to paraphrase Pascal, reason knows the heart that reason does not understand.

From Virgil and Ignatius of Loyola to Albert Einstein many intellectual geniuses have proclaimed the value of inner experience and imaginative involvement. But only those who give themselves permission to look foolish in their own eyes and experience a new way of using their mind for self-awareness will feel comfortable enough to employ this method with their clients.

5

Personal Experience

By experiential psychotherapy I mean *the applied theory of human transformation emphasizing its process or the experiences had in the existential trajectory from being in one mode to being in another, better mode.* Among the experiential therapists I count a mixture of distant cousins who do not even know they are related: gestaltists, existentialists, bioenergists and Reichians, logotherapists and focusing therapists, primal screamers, psychodramatists, brief therapy practitioners of the Mental Research Institute of Palo Alto, and many more who live within the humanistic-existential atmosphere. Although their theories differ vastly, from psychoanalytical to behavioral goal orientations, their basic method is experiential. Human transformation is produced (at least in theory) *through a new and truer experience of self*; not through understanding and insight, not through a passive reception of behavioral variables, not through blind obedience to prescriptions imposed by the therapist. Mahrer (1983) stated it thus: ''It is a family of psychotherapies rooted in the humanistic-existential theory of human beings and accepting experiencing as its pivotal axis of psychotherapeutic change'' (p. 45).

In the terms used throughout this book, we could identify experiential therapies as those which are more concerned with right-hemispheric functioning in the process of human transformation than other therapies. But since experience is mainly a perceptual reality, imagination can be used as the main means of experiencing. The often quoted statement by Epictetus, ''What disturbs men's minds is not events but their judgments on events," implies people's imaginative experiencing. What occurs is filtered, interpreted, colored, by one's "judgment" or mental activity, which always includes imagination. Here is where hypnosis enters. Though a legitimate relative of the experiential cousins, hypnosis lived in exile until fairly recently. The fact that hypnosis is 200 years old does not make it close to the other therapies, because it was not in the mainstream of the better known approaches to human change. The New Hypnosis is eminently experiential, paying attention to bodily sensations as a means of integrating conscious and subconscious elements of the personality.

In this chapter, the experiential aspects of *negative self-hypnosis* as a means to understanding noneffective conduct will be examined. Then, the importance of *self-hypnosis* as an essential experiential part of the New Hypnosis will be discussed. Finally, in accordance with the applied and practical trend of this book, I shall address myself to *the client-therapist interaction* from the experiential point of view.

NEGATIVE SELF-HYPNOSIS (NSH)

This concept and its designation were introduced by me in 1981 and further elaborated in one of my books (1982a). At this point, a fresher look at NSH will help us realize that it is closely related to the concept of the self-fulfilling prophecies. These are hypnotic in nature, namely, *accepted self-suggestions or beliefs put into action nonconsciously*. I will also relate my NSH concept to Blumenthal's (1984) important work on self-suggestion in order to tie it later to his Rational Suggestion Therapy.

Self-fulfilling Prophecies

At the core of such events lies belief. Faith can "move mountains" to make one's path through life easier or to crush one with their mass. Watzlawick (1984) defines a self-fulfilling prophecy as "an assumption or prediction that, purely as a result of having been made, causes the expected or predicted event to occur and thus confirms its own 'accuracy'" (p. 95). This is a definition of the self-fulfilling prochecy's effect, not of its process. But further on Watzlawick focuses on the latter: "*Only when a prophecy is believed*, that is, only when it is seen as a fact that has, so to speak, already happened in the future, can it have a tangible effect on the present and thereby fulfill itself. Where *this element of belief or conviction* is absent, this effect will be absent as well" (p. 100) (my emphasis).

People experience themselves nongenuinely through their expectations. These expectations (beliefs, convictions) are often held and defended consciously, although their formation in people's minds is nonconscious. Watzlawick (1984), referring to the philosopher Karl Popper's (1974) comments on *Oedipus Rex*, explains this conscious-subconscious reality. Oedipus' parents, *because they believed* the oracle, took extraordinary steps to protect him from killing his father and marrying his mother. In spending so much energy trying to protect themselves from the destiny *they had believed in*, they made it happen. Had Oedipus' parents ignored the oracle, ridiculed it and gone about their own business, the prophecy never would have been fulfilled. Oedipus believed the oracle, too. If someone had asked him, "Why are you running away?" he would have had a perfectly rational explanation: to avoid the oracle's prediction. But the fact that he *believed* the oracle to begin with was the nonconscious element that contributed to the formation of the self-fulfilling prophecy.

This is what NSH is all about: a nonconscious belief which influences actions in much the same way as a post-hypnotic suggestion. If asked why we do this, we have a logical, conscious answer but we don't realize we are acting under the powerful influence of a nonconscious conviction.

In Chapter 7, I shall refer to the power of the mind to heal, or rather to accelerate and facilitate the healing processes. The beneficial effects of placebos come only from the patient's mind: the belief that this "medication" will produce healing, even though the "medication" is a chemically inert substance (see Benson and Epstein, 1975). But the same mind that heals can kill.

When the beliefs that control our actions are negative, as in poor Oedipus' case, we are under the influence of our own NSH. The New Hypnosis helps clients to uncover the NSH at work in their lives. A key initial question to ask the client when in hypnosis is, What's happening inside of you when you project yourself into your future? This, or a variation of it, can apply to any presenting problem. When the image or mental projection of the self-fulfilling prophecy is encouraged, its magic disappears. The client recognizes the subconscious messages and, with the help of the therapist, unmasks them first, in order to substitute them for self-chosen, constructive operating principles. This process is exemplified in the 28-year-old man who kept saying he did not want to be like his father who had died a few months before at 61 years of age, after making many enemies. The father had been a ruthless businessman who owned a successful chain of stores. However, his success had been at the expense of many people and through innumerable injustices inflicted on practically everybody who had dealings with him. The son's relationship with his father had been strained and explosive. The former had preferred to be rather poor and independent from his father than well-off but under his influence and control. Now that he was dead, the son had been even more concerned than previously with not being like his father. He had rationalized his posture but, to his surprise, he was feeling depressed. In hypnosis he became aware of his tremendous fear of being like his father. He also recognized that he had many traits like his father and that he was obsessed with this issue. Chapter 9 will present this case in detail. Here I merely want to point out that these realizations "dehypnotized" him from his NSH and broke the spell of his disguised self-fulfilling prophecy, which was that his personality traits, like those of his father, would overtake him and that he would become like him. All this was accomplished by his personal "experiencing." Argumentation, reasons, logic, and other left-hemispheric activities were not used. But thanks to the active imaginative involvement through the New Hypnosis method the young man was able first to fully accept the personality traits in him which were like those of his father. He experienced himself as being that which he consciously was denying and avoiding. This new experience allowed him, next, to dismiss in a free, choosing manner those traits he did not like, even though they were his own. He confronted his fear by seeing himself as the ugly picture he despised. Then he was able to decide not to be like his father in spite of his own "liability" and to take action in order to become what he wanted to become. It is also important to note that all this material came up during the first session, elicited by the projection into the future which he experienced when he was in hypnosis.

Self-suggestions

It might be clinically beneficial always to look for the NSH, assuming that it *is* there as a negative suggestion which has been accepted nonconsciously. This can be further understood thanks to Blumenthal's (1984) elaboration of the work of the New Nancy school. In Chapter 1 spontaneous suggestions were mentioned. A refinement of these are *conditional spontaneous autosuggestions* (Baudouin, 1922): behaviors elicited each time certain conditions occur. This phenomenon was first restricted to physical ailments, and the theory was that probably the first time the negative reaction happened it was due to a true physical malfunction. Subsequently, the same reaction took place spontaneously, triggered solely by *the strong expectation of the symptom*. And Blumenthal (1984) explains: "An idea learned from prior experience had been employed without conscious deliberation when triggered by key conditions similar to the original experience. With each subsequent experience, the autosuggestion became more and more part of the event, and soon an entrenched habit was formed" (p. 58).

If we analyze human problems within their circumstances or "conditions," we find this mechanism at work. In this sense, the behavioral concepts of reinforcement and conditioning can be understood more fully and humanistically by applying the principle of conditional spontaneous autosuggestion. The *conditions* become the stimulus, while the response is *the result of the learned autosuggestions.* If this is the case, the aim of our work shifts from changing behavior to that of changing beliefs and learned self-suggestions, since the unprofitable self-suggestions have to be substituted by new freely chosen ones. In the words of Blumenthal (1984): "It is desirable to attempt to alter unprofitable autosuggestion with rationally developed autosuggestion in advance of anticipated conditions. This technique may be used for the immense benefit of the individual whose current ideas are working against his/her own best interest" (p. 58). To accomplish this aim, Blumenthal proposes *rational suggestion therapy* (RST) whose aim "is to master autosuggestion by using the therapy arena to enable the individual to control the source of autosuggestion" (p. 58) which, for him, is the conscious self. Based on this he proposes three phases for RST: first, to choose consciously to change the unproductive idea (the *theoretical phase*). Second, the *practical phase*, in order to implant the new ideas in the subconscious by means of New Hypnosis techniques and, finally, the *spontaneous phase*, which is what happens to the individual next time the adverse conditions appear. The last phase, obviously, is the measure of success of the treatment. Blumenthal's (1984) three phases are a practical method to undo the damage of NSH. It exemplifies the experiential nature of the New Hypnosis to the point that the new behavior in phase three is a manifestation of a real inner transformation. In this approach, also, intellectual analysis, the historical search for the "whys" of the problem leading to understanding and insight, is absent. But the vivid experience of a new self is at the core of Rational Suggestion Therapy.

SELF-HYPNOSIS

In the New Hypnosis the client does the work, not the therapist. Elsewhere (Araoz, 1982a), I have commented on the important contributions of Diamond (1982b) and Katz (1979) to the experiential aspects of self-hypnosis. Others, like Tossi, Reardon, and Rudy (1977), Goba (1979) and Miller (1981), for example, have done effective work of their own with self-hypnosis. But more than the rest, Fromm and her associates (1981) collected important research-based information on the nature, characteristics, and applicability of self-hypnosis. From this wealth of material, the conclusion about the experiential essence of self-hypnosis is inescapable. Clients experience themselves differently while practicing self-hypnosis; they are rehearsing for the new, richer, and truer self they are striving to become. If we take Miller's (1981) process therapy as an example, the core of it is the directed imagery practice of his "ideal real self." Self-hypnosis consists of practicing imagery-modeling of this real self in the different social circumstances (with outcomes according to the patient's wishes) which previously elicited undesirable behavior. This self-hypnosis practice acclimates clients to a new modality of being, and allows them to become whom they want to be, because they are experiencing themselves in a different way—as capable, feeling the pride in their ability to cope and master.

Nearly all books on hypnosis have a section on self-hypnosis (e.g., Shaw, 1977), and articles about it appear frequently in the journals (e.g., Gross, 1984) or even in popular magazines (e.g., Hunt, 1984). Self-hypnosis is popular but it is often presented as a gimmicky procedure, almost separated from and independent of everything we know about hypnosis in general. The New Hypnosis presents to clients all hypnosis as self-hypnosis, following T. X. Barber's (in press) reasoning: 1) It avoids or at least minimizes many fears associated with hypnosis; 2) it emphasizes calmness and inner peace rather than the bizarre phenomena attributed to hypnosis by the media; 3) it places control in the hands of the client; 4) it allows therapists of any school to be themselves rather than to attempt a procedure with which they might not be comfortable; and 5) it gives therapists flexibility in using hypnosis, maximizing the feedback from clients. By flexibility T. X. Barber (in press) means the possibility of entering self-hypnosis with the client or of communicating with the client after having entered self-hypnosis. I shall return to this issue in the next section of this chapter.

By presenting hypnotic work as self-hypnosis, the therapist

conveys several important messages. The implication is: 1) that this will be the therapist's and client's unique, personal, individualized experience; 2) that the therapist does not have any sure-proof method to make things happen, and consequently, the client and the therapist have to find the best means to enter self-hypnosis and to benefit from it; and 3) that this mind activity is a natural procedure the person has to learn through practice. Frequently I find myself using the analogy of running. It is a natural activity but people who have not run for many years have to learn with progressive practice what are their optimum levels (speed, time, distance) and that they cannot be expert runners after just a few times of doing it. Practice will make even an older healthy adult a good runner, even though he or she had never run before. So, too, with self-hypnosis.

However, I do not introduce hypnosis to clients formally. Hypnosis is *the* modus operandi if one is willing to accept it. I tell clients that *this therapy is rooted in experiencing oneself differently*, not in talking (Zilbergeld, 1983). This is especially necessary to emphasize with clients who have familiarity with traditional therapy. I make it clear that my main function is to help them *change* and that I do not have any solid, scientific evidence to believe that talk, leading to insight, necessarily produces change. In their classic study on human change, Watzlawick, Weakland, and Fisch (1974) mention the "more of the same" phenomenon, when the solution becomes the problem. Often in traditional therapy, when years of talk, supposedly leading to insight in order to produce change, have not accomplished this, the prescription is more of the same. And clients—strangely enough—buy this wholeheartedly. When these "experienced" clients are exposed to the New Hypnosis, they need some time to diminish the talking and increase the experiencing during the therapy sessions.

There is a special problem with patients who are referred for hypnosis. In this case, because often they expect "to be out of it" or fear it or have fantastic expectations of the magical power of hypnosis, the above reference to *self-hypnosis*, rather than to *hypnosis*, is especially helpful.

Gestalt Therapy

A few words on Gestalt therapy are in order. People often ask me if what I do is not Gestalt therapy and, if so, why I insist on referring to the New Hypnosis. If the primary tool and goal of Gestalt therapy are "awareness" or being in touch with one's own being at the present moment (Simkin, 1979) or Gestalt *is* the awareness continuum (L. Perls, 1973), how does this differ from "experiencing" and right-hemispheric activity which are the trademarks of the New Hypnosis? "Gestalt therapy views the entire biopsychosocial field, including organism/environment, as important" (Yontef, quoted in Applebaum, 1976, p. 763). How is this different from the attention to somatics in the OLD C model proposed in Chapter 4? The comparisons could continue to be listed. The main point to be made is that the New Hypnosis is not a school of psychotherapy with its own theory of personality and psychopathology, as Gestalt therapy is. The New Hypnosis is a convenient and flexible way of applying hypnotic principles by psychotherapists of any theoretical orientation. In the actual process of psychotherapy, however, and the techniques used, I personally become very "Gestaltist," and humbly give credit and thanks to the Gestalt school. However, by not being labeled a Gestalt therapist I am free to do many things in the clinical setting which do not agree with their pure theory, such as using direct suggestions. But other New Hypnosis practitioners such as Erickson (Rossi, 1980), T. X. Barber (in press), and Blumenthal (1984) are not close to the Gestalt modality in their clinical work.

"Awareness" in itself can be curative, as Fritz Perls (1976) believed, and because of this theoretical position I help clients identify with what happens in *their* here and now. I use the New Hypnosis to help them recognize and accept their "world," and act according to this "reality" with all its ramifications. Only at this existential juncture can a person decide to be one or another aspect of the self. Beisser (1970) put it well in terms of the conflict between what one *should be* and what one *thinks* he *is*, "never fully identifying with either" (p. 78). The New Hypnosis, as I use it, resolves the conflict by helping clients own completely all aspects of their being and then choose which ones they want to keep.

One thing is certain: There is no antagonism between Gestalt therapy and the New Hypnosis. As a matter of fact, many Gestalt techniques are hypnotic in nature. Think of the intervention where the client is asked to imagine someone who is not physically present (the person may have died a long time ago) and address himself to her. To do this successfully, the client has to be in a hypnotic frame of mind or trance and the intensity of affect indicates, at that time, the measure of the hypnotic experience. But this is at the level of techniques. Gestalt therapy, in the words of Levitsky and Simkin (1972) "contains a philosophy of growth, of healthy human functioning; it is essentially a philosophy of being," whereas the New Hypnosis, as such, remains at the level of techniques, making it possible for therapists of diverse philosophies to employ it.

CLIENT-THERAPIST INTERACTION

The flesh and blood of hypnosis—its multidimensional clinical richness and variation—only appears *when hypnosis is viewed in terms of the dynamic interrelationships between real people*. (Shor, 1959, p. 601)

These words unlock the door to a reality uniquely pertaining to hypnosis. However, few people have opened that door. Diamond (1982b; 1983b) proceeded equipped partly with psychodynamic principles (like the few since Shor who preceded him, e.g., Field, 1979), and distinguished four relational dimensions in hypnosis, as I shall discuss presently. On the other hand, Mahrer (1983) assumed "that the personhood or identity of the therapist can assimilate into or fuse with the personhood or identity of the patient . . . that patient and therapist exist in multiple phenomenal worlds constructed by the patient, the therapist and both conjointly" (p. 145). I shall briefly review these two positions, that of Diamond and that of Mahrer, in order to focus on the experiential nature of the New Hypnosis concerning the client-therapist interaction.

Diamond (1983a) explained the four relational dimensions he discovered in hypnosis. These are *hypnotic transference, hypnotic working alliance, hypnotic fusional alliance,* and *hypnotic real relationship.* The first relational dimension frequently starts long before the patient meets the hypnotherapist and may produce the "hypnotic transference neurosis," as Morris and Gardner (1959) called it. Hypnotic transference occurs when ancient parent-child elements emerge or when there is regression to the Oedipal situation projected onto the hypnotherapist.

The second relational dimension, according to Diamond (1983a), has both irrational and reality-oriented aspects. On the latter side is the *adaptive regression* of Gill and Brenman (1959) or *the regression in the service of the ego* of Kris (1952), so that there always remains an unhypnotized observing ego. On the irrational side of the working alliance, Diamond followed Nunberg (1948) who speculated that the client idealizes the hypnotherapist, then finds comfort in that ideal, and thus permits the hypnotherapist to influence him. However, the irrational elements of this alliance are therapeutic and positive, often fostered by the therapist. This is the reason to call this a working or therapeutic alliance.

The third relational dimension in hypnosis—fusional or narcissistic—consists of "the subject's identification with the hypnotist's (real or presumed) characteristics *at a bodily-level,* and participating in the 'magic,' charisma, or whatever the hypnotist evokes" (Diamond, 1983a, p. 28) (my emphasis). It is speculated that this takes place at an oral, pre-Oedipal, narcissistic level and that it produces a condition of artificial symbiosis or fusion. Finally, the *hypnotic real relationship* refers to such elements as mutual concern and respect between therapist and client.

Before drawing some practical conclusions I would like to turn to Mahrer's (1983) ideas. He claimed that "the therapist-patient role relationship truncates the amount of sheer attention the patient can place upon internal personality processes" (p. 166), which means that as long as the patient's attention is on the therapist, very little can be deployed onto the patient's own internal personality processes. Does this mean that when a patient is interacting with the therapist it is possible for the patient to ignore the presence of the therapist? Of course not, but Mahrer's (1983) point is that talking to each other, the interaction that takes place between therapist and client in traditional, nonexperiential therapy, is precisely the reason why most therapy is useless: It distracts the client from his internal processes; it cuts short the patient's relation with his current inner experience; it remains left-hemispheric. Patient-therapist interaction as a focus is a distraction from experiencing oneself genuinely: "to the extent therapist and patient talk to one another about it (i.e., the latter's problems) the patient is unable to have a relation with it. The patient is thereby unable to see it fully, confront or engage it, perceive and grasp it, encounter it, feel it, experience it" (pp. 166–167).

Referring to Naranjo (1969) and May (1958), Mahrer (1983) underlined the common error of assuming that therapist acceptance of the client will automatically help the client experience his own being. Indeed, emphasis on patient-therapist issues deemphasizes "the relationship between the patient and genuinely internal personality processes" (p. 167). Even worse, such emphasis may only validate the separateness of many patients from their internal personality processes.

Consequences

The implications of the client-therapist interaction are many but I am especially interested in its experiential aspects. In general, the relationship with another person during hypnosis facilitates awareness, self-discovery, and being in touch with areas of the self previously ignored or distorted, as Sullivan (1953) explained about psychotherapy in general. However, this happens only if the interaction is enhancing not just for the client, but also for the therapist. This presupposes a relation between equals at the essential level of humanness. Attempts at attaining this goal of human equality are not uncommon. For instance, T. X. Barber (in press) joins the client in the trance or, more accurately, enters trance when the client does, in his attempt to facilitate self-hypnosis in the other person. Mahrer (1983) also participates during the session in experiences similar to those of the client. Diamond (1980, 1982a) goes a step further, inviting the client to hypnotize him as a means of furthering hypnotherapy in certain special situations.

This relation among equals at the essential level of awareness has some important implications, fitting within the OLD C model proposed in the previous chapter. First, it is a humble realization on the part of the therapist that he does not have the answers to the client's questions. He "leads" the client to find the answers which exist in the subconscious or which, through the experiential process of the New Hypnosis, are formed and emerge. The therapist's expertise lies at this technical level: He is the expert in guiding the client into his inner personality processes.

The second implication, coming from the previous overview of the relational aspect in psychotherapy generally and in hypnotherapy in particular, is that the focus of attention must be on the client's inner processes and current psychic experiences, not on the relationship between client and therapist. The relationship is merely the facilitating environment for the process of self-discovery to take place. The focus on the relationship is never therapeutic in and of itself. It is only justified when the current inner experience of the client involves the therapist in some way.

A corollary of the above is that the hypnotherapist cannot just be himself (another myth frequently advocated as therapeutic) but must be highly disciplined *not* to be himself. He must adhere scrupulously to his role of guide. He cannot lose sight of his role of facilitator for the client's awareness of inner realities unconsciously ignored, denied, distorted, or repressed. The hypnotherapist must be *his professional self*; and his private self must stay out of the therapeutic situation as much as possible.

Of course, there is nothing new here. Psychoanalysts require this aseptic attitude on the basis of not contaminating the transference. Good therapists, regardless of their theories or philosophies, have realized long ago that client and therapist are equals at the human level of existence (with all their uncertainties and doubts, hopes and dreams, finiteness and vulnerability, joys and loves), but the moment they enter into the therapeutic "contract," the role of the hypnotherapist must be clearly and fully assumed.

This unambiguous stance is the unique experience of any good therapy for the client. This is especially true in hypnotherapy where exquisite sensitivity to the use of one's words is even more essential than in other, left-hemispheric therapies. And the clear role of the therapist is even more important in the New Hypnosis which starts with an almost worshipful observation of the client's language style, important statements, and somatics. This observation is not in order to make sense of these elements of behavior, to analyze them or to interpret them, but simply to lead the client to an inner, full, true experience and awareness of what is happening inside of him at the moment, and of which those three basic behaviors are external manifestations. In this sense the New Hypnosis is experiential for the client because he has during hypnotherapy the unique experience of entering into new territories of his self, discovering aspects of himself heretofore unknown. Because of this experience, he expands his psychological being, and in so doing he also takes possession of new aspects of his physical being. The latter happens, at the simplest level, when clients learn to relax. In many cases a client achieves great physical feats, such as control of pain, even to the extent of undergoing surgery with hypnosis as sole anesthesia.

CONCLUSION

The New Hypnosis takes a humbler posture than Traditional Hypnosis, with its concern for scientific objectivity and measurement of hypnotizability and depth, scales, scores, and statistics. This more modest position of the New Hypnosis is in harmony with a development emerging even in the most exact of sciences. Traditional Hypnosis went with the times, with the old science started by Copernicus, which naively believed it could understand the cosmos, measure it, control it, dominate and subjugate it for man's ends. "Modern science" became the goddess of the world and was worshipped as such. Now, after three centuries, scientists are still puzzled; they confess their perplexity, suspecting that the key to the understanding of the universe is the human person. The razor-sharp distinction between objective and subjective reality may have become as obsolete as Copernican physics after relativity and quantum mechanics—in science, yes, and in hypnosis.

Thus, the New Hypnosis becomes less "scientific," and more naturalistic, spontaneous, and experiential. Being is experience. The New Hypnosis facilitates one's personal experience of self, cuts through the layers of negative self-hypnosis which led us to think we knew who we were, even though we were submerged in falsehood. It helps us change our set beliefs to a new openness, to the evolving, changing, flow which is life, to participate more fully in our *becoming* through experiencing.

We, as the experts practicing the New Hypnosis, turn into humble guides and facilitators of that *process* and, because of it, encourage what others may label "unreal" or "nonsense." Thus, we establish that therapeutic alliance which, because it is an alliance, modifies us also, expands our being, and allows us to join the dance of existence.

This is why it takes a special effort to enter the frame of mind of the New Hypnosis. It is similar to the Zen attitude of receptivity and openness, the attitude of *the beginner's mind*, as Suzuki (1970), the founder of the first Zen center in this country, claimed. Such a mind is devoid of absolute certainties, always questioning, searching, and never closed; it is a mind that questions the obvious, the real and rational, what is common sense and self-evident. The New Hypnosis makes an inflexible demand on its practitioners: to have a beginner's mind all the time. This is what is hidden in the first step of the OLD C model. Observation means to have a beginner's mind so that interaction with the client does not stop, interrupt, or distort the client's experience.

As I conclude this chapter on the experiential nature of the New Hypnosis, I am struck by the paradox of the theory of non-theory. Much as I try to convince myself that the New Hypnosis is a method or technology and not a theory, the more I delve into it, the closer I come to a theoretical position: the quantum logic, as opposed to classical logic. With the ideal of a beginner's mind, I must accept it, knowing that this is only another step into mythos, as opposed to logos. The New Hypnosis is a state of being, indescribable. It can only be experienced, and, as practitioners of the New Hypnosis, *we* must experience it, both in ourselves and for ourselves, before guiding and facilitating the experience of our clients.

Part III

New Directions

The field of hypnosis is becoming more and more exciting with every passing month. Books, articles, and conferences point to new areas of applicability. During the XXIII Olympics in Los Angeles, for example, the popular press was bringing to the public's attention the important role of hypnosis (called either imagery, or psychovisualization, or inner-mind techniques) in the training of the athletic teams.

Although a whole book could be written on the new directions hypnosis is taking currently, I have chosen Family Therapy and Healing for subjective reasons. My doctoral degree from Columbia University is in family counseling, and family therapy has been a constant interest of mine for the last 25 years. It is exciting to see that recently more and more papers and books are appearing on the application of hypnosis to this field. Chapter 6 is an overview of concepts and methods to use hypnosis effectively with families.

I have also long been fascinated by the area of healing, having been active in the American Society of Psychosomatic Dentistry and Medicine for many years, and more recently, in the International Psychosomatics Institute, as well as in the editorial work of the *International Journal of Psychosomatics*. Because the evidence keeps mounting that semantic input is decoded as somatic output, I have tried to provide an overview of what is known today, while also presenting my own approach with clients referred with psychosomatic problems.

91

6

Family Hypnotherapy

This chapter, born from my interest in family therapy, will present a discussion and review of what I like to call Family Hypnotherapy. The review shall comprise different ways of using hypnosis and hypnotic principles with families in particular and with a systemic orientation in general, as well as my own application of the New Hypnosis to human systems, specifically to the family. In so doing I shall present clinical vignettes, though one of the families mentioned in this chapter will receive special and detailed attention in Chapter 8.

The use of hypnosis in family situations is not new. Erickson (Haley, 1973) treated many families with hypnosis, if by "family" we include problems centered on family members, especially spouses, and unresolved problems with one's family of origin. Haley's (1973) *Uncommon Therapy* is a book on family therapy using the New Hypnosis, where he describes in detail, often in Erickson's own words, the latter's procedures. However, he often worked with one family member, not with the whole group.

Many others have employed hypnosis in family cases, as a cursory review of the literature shows. Most of these hypnotic interventions in family therapy fall under the category of the New Hypnosis. For instance, Morrison (1981) proposes imagery techniques "to recreate the sensorial surroundings of childhood" (p. 53), concluding that "the memory of such events often produces the kind of rich imagery which elicits strong feelings about a parent" (ibid.). He also employs imagery techniques to produce sig-

nificant breakthroughs with married couples; one effective method is to picture ''one's spouse standing next to the opposite sex
parent and to note the similarities and differences of both persons''
(ibid.). Lovern and Zohn (1982) employ Ericksonian methods in
multiple family group therapy with alcoholics. Their techniques
include unconscious conditioning (Erickson and Rossi, 1979), psychological shock (Erickson et al., 1976), indirect suggestion and
therapeutic bind (Erickson and Rossi, 1979). The Lanktons (1982)
also use indirect suggestions and binds in family therapy, with
such comments as: ''You can either learn from this experience
or teach it to your children''; ''Your conscious mind didn't know
that your unconscious would choose the right thing to begin therapy, but your conscious mind could wonder which topic your
unconscious would choose''; or again, ''You may learn from the
experience or merely use the experience.'' The Lanktons' book
(1983) is interspersed with innumerable ways of using the New
Hypnosis with couples and families.

Although in family therapy nonformal hypnosis is frequently found, more traditional hypnotic approaches are also employed. Thus Goba (1978) proposed many formal hypnosis techniques to help couples communicate effectively. Braun (1978),
taking a psychoanalytical orientation, introduced important hypnotic interventions with families, always helping parents and children *to experience* their family situation differently, rather than
to merely analyze, understand, and make logical sense of what
is happening. In a limited research, I studied the effects of formal hypnosis on 12 couples who were in couples group therapy
(Araoz, 1979). Every three months new goals were established
(improved verbal communication, cooperative child-rearing, and
improved sexual functioning), simultaneously alternating hypnotic and nonhypnotic methods in order to attain them. During
the 18 months of the study, the hypnotic techniques consistent-
ly proved more effective. Earlier, I (Araoz, 1978) had studied traditional hypnotic methods in conjoint couple therapy.

More recently, other hypnotic realities in family interaction
have been investigated by Jaffe (1980), Ritterman (1983), and
Calof (1985), among others. These three authors focus on nega-

tive effects of hypnotic influences among family members. These effects can range from physical illness, as Minuchin (1974; Minuchin, Baker & Rosman, 1978) demonstrated, to "craziness" in communication. Both Jaffe (1980) and Ritterman (1983) use the negative hypnosis at work in dysfunctional families as a stepping stone towards a constructive use of hypnotic techniques.

There is obviously much to be understood about *family hypnotherapy*. Therefore, this chapter will investigate first the traditional application of hypnosis with families. Then the indirect and nontraditional forms will be presented, demonstrating use of the New Hypnosis, and including special reference to two recent noteworthy contributions. Finally, my own approach to family hypnotherapy will be summarized.

It should be emphasized that nobody without formal training in family therapy, no matter with how much knowledge and expertise in hypnosis, should get involved in family work. The innumerable dynamics between family members, spanning from past to present to future psychological realities, are too complex for amateurs.

TRADITIONAL APPLICATIONS OF HYPNOSIS WITH FAMILIES

Psychodynamic principles prevail in this method of using hypnosis with families. The focus is on introjects and projections, following Framo (1972), Boszormenyi-Nagy (1965), and other object relations authors. Perhaps the best representative of this group is Braun (1978, 1984). He (1978) outlined the five phases of hypnotic work with families. These are: 1) induction; 2) deepening; 3) work; 4) termination; and 5) processing. He states that "hypnosis is a series of semi-formalized procedures to heighten awareness and suggestibility through mental training" (p. 7). He starts with a prehypnotic interview in which he creates a mental and physical environment conducive to hypnosis. By this he means that he will ask people to change chairs "to separate combatants or place someone very anxious near someone of comfort" (p. 10). Using Kramer's (1968) typology, he conceptualizes four main family styles: the *conflictual* (open fighting); the *over/under-adequate* (one-up or one-down positions in the family: one member is symptomatic while the others appear symptom-free but when the symptom-bearer gets better, the family experiences strain); the *united front* (overly harmonious); and the *mixed* type (the most common).

Hypnosis is then used to help create a new framework. First, it can be useful to give the family a shared pleasurable experience of relaxation, which serves to build a common foundation and trust. Hypnorelaxation is, then, a general technique. The choice of other techniques depends on the therapist's imagination and clinical experience. Braun (1978) lists several. The *reverse blink technique* asks the family

> to start with their eyes closed and to open and shut them quickly each time I count a number. Suggestions are made between counts for deeper relaxation that eventually the eyes will remain closed while deeper relaxation is attained with each count. Different members will stop opening their eyes at different times, but eventually all will be relaxed with their eyes closed. At this point other fantasy work can be accomplished. (p. 19)

Braun also proposes the use of projective hypnotic techniques with families in order to relive and review past incidents so the reaction to them can become more effective.

Age regression is another hypnotic technique which can be beneficial for the family to relive, explore, and resolve past events which are still "unfinished." Though Braun (1984) does not mention it specifically, age progression is another traditional hypnotic technique which prepares the family to either face a difficult situation, such as the hospitalization of one member, or find better ways of interacting and enjoying themselves as a family group.

The application of traditional hypnotic techniques in family therapy is flexible. A therapist can work with one family member in trance, involving the others at appropriate times; similarly, he can work with a marital couple either alone or in the family setting, though for a couple's sexual problems, the other family members are usually excluded.

Regarding specific applications of these techniques, the *over/underadequate* family can be helped by the use of the ideal self. In Braun's (1984) words, one of the family members

> is asked to create a mental image of himself, not as he is today, but as he would like to be. Ask the patient to describe the image and hold it in memory for later. Then ask him to create an image of himself as he perceives himself today. In reality the patient is somewhere between these two descriptions; getting this feedback from family members is therapeutic. The therapist can also ask the patient to merge these two fantasized images by having them face each other, walk toward each other and merge into one person. The patient often gains a sense of mastery and freedom to act after this. (p. 334)

For the *conflictual* family, an imaginary projection of how the family members could interact in a specific situation conflict-free becomes a goal towards which they all can aim. In the case of the *united front* family, a fantasy situation (such as a space flight) which requires collaboration among its members is created. How they handle in fantasy unexpected situations of stress helps the therapist and the family members themselves understand strengths, fears, and other dynamics.

In all these descriptions of Traditional Hypnosis, it is interesting to note that the hypnotic work does not follow rigid patterns. The moment hypnosis is used outside the one-to-one situation, it becomes more flexible and naturalistic, even for workers like Braun, who is adapting traditional techniques of individual hypnosis to a new setting, namely, family therapy. The focus in this approach is on the intrapsychic realities as they are reflected in the family interaction.

INDIRECT AND NON-TRADITIONAL HYPNOSIS WITH FAMILIES

This approach attempts to expand, on the one hand, the traditional use of hypnosis, which is centered on the individual, extending it to the family system. On the other hand, it also tries

to expand the systemic outlook by paying attention to and working with the interpsychic realities in families. It is an attempt at
integrating systemic and psychodynamic theories. This integration, however, is not a way of reverting to what traditional therapies believe, that insight leads to change, but is consistent with
the Ericksonian belief in *change leading to insight*. Calof (1985)
quoted Erickson as saying that Jay Haley brings the whole family
to therapy in order to change, while he (Erickson) was content
to see the symptom-bearer, so that by changing him or her the
whole family had to change in its way of relating to the symptom-
bearer-without-the-symptom.

Systemic advocates have often rejected intrapsychic dynamics
as if they were fictions of Freud and his disciples. In so doing,
they have become as dogmatic and inflexible as those whom they
oppose. Family hypnotherapists using the New Hypnosis are expanding the view of family interaction to its real boundaries,
which include both systemic *and* intrapsychic events. In this area
we find many remarkable contributions. To appreciate them fully,
we must be perceptive of hypnotic maneuvers even in those who
do not practice hypnosis as such. For example, paradoxical therapists, such as Madanes (1981), understand the origin and maintenance of a child's dysfunctional behavior as a help or protection within the family system. The child, "hypnotized" by the
family structure, perpetuates a behavior which keeps the neurotic
family system alive. Selvini Palazzoli and her co-workers (1978,
1980) move families away from left-hemispheric functioning and
make it impossible for them not to switch to right-hemispheric
activity by means of paradox and counterparadox. The clients,
fixated in dysfunctional behavior, are seen as hypnotized by the
rules they have established for themselves without realizing it.
To quote (Selvini Palazzoli et al., 1978): "The power is only in
the rules of the game which cannot be changed by the people
involved in it" (p. 6). The people involved in the game (or mental frame of reference) believe (in a negative self-hypnotic way)
that this is the only way they can be. What Selvini Palazzoli and
her co-workers do is, indeed, to dehypnotize them or rather to
change their crystalized frame of reference into alternate ones.

Weeks and L'Abate (1982) have listed the five principles of paradoxical intervention, which are all related to hypnotic concepts as I understand and have explained them in the first part of this book.

Principle One: New symptoms are positively relabeled, reframed or connoted. . . .
Principle Two: The symptom is linked to the other members of the system. . . .
Principle Three: Reverse the symptom's vector. . . .
Principle Four: Prescribe and sequence paradoxical interventions over time in order to bind off the reappearance of the symptom. . . .
Principle Five: The paradoxical prescription must force the clients to act on the task in some way. (pp. 90–92)

The first two principles address themselves to reversing the process of negative self-hypnosis (Araoz, 1981, 1982a) so that the negative connotations of the symptom are minimized. First, *its functional role* is uncovered. By so doing, the problem starts to be viewed differently. An alternate reality emerges. Emphasis is also placed on *the system* which the symptom intends to serve (or on the system for which the symptom started and exists). This second principle stresses what Ritterman (1983) has masterfully described as a form of mutual hypnosis which takes place among family members. I shall return to Ritterman's contributions later in this chapter.

The third principle is concerned with control. The family system is not helpless in face of the symptom. By deliberate production of the symptom either as to its frequency or intensity, the symptomatic person or family *controls* the symptom and stops feeling helpless about it. Weeks and L'Abate (1982) suggest two basic ways to reverse the symptom within the family system. The first is to encourage family members to foster the symptom of the symptom-bearer. The second is to teach the other family members to act paradoxically. An example taken from Weeks and L'Abate (1982) may help clarify this. If the problem in a family is a daughter who struggles to control the mother, the former

is asked to do this even more intently, while the latter is instructed to act in a helpless and childlike manner with the daughter.
The hypnotic nature of acting *as if* the daughter were in charge
and the mother were a helpless child creates alternate realities
in the whole system which, by that very measure, is forced to
change and to seek a new equilibrium.

According to the fourth and fifth principles, both forms of post-
hypnotic suggestion, the therapist follows a strategy which includes positive reframing and symptom prescription, predicting
a reoccurrence of the problem and prescribing the relapse. The
client's active involvement is obtained either by some prescribed
ritual of a paradoxical nature or by setting things up so that when
something concretely determined and known to occur happens,
the symptom will appear. Examples follow.

The wife, who could not trust her husband's protestations of
love after having found out that he had seen another woman,
was told that she was right because he felt guilty and needed
punishment. In hypnosis she was encouraged to go over all the
ways in which she could punish him by refusing to cook for him,
to do his laundry, to go out with him, by spending much more
than usual so that he had to work harder, etc. The result of this
thought experiment came from her, without any help from her
husband or me. She concluded that this was ridiculous; either
she wanted the marriage or not; either she was with him or not.
Therefore she was going to try to trust him and to give the marriage another chance, making this a new beginning.

Bobby was an 11-year-old bright boy who was doing very poorly in school. The mother, trying "to help him," got into the habit
of yelling at him, telling him how much this hurt her, and so
forth, which only helped to upset Bobby, damaging even more
his concentration to do homework. The mother was told not to
help Bobby with his homework unless Joe, the husband, was
home. She was to spend exactly 15 minutes with Joe before helping Bobby with homework. During these 15 minutes she would
tell Joe how frustrated she was, how unfair this was, how bad
Bobby was to her, etc. She had to do this for exactly 15 minutes,
timed by Joe to the second. The result was that she refused to

help Bobby with his homework. Bobby was then asked to work on it alone and to request help from his father only when he *really* needed it and only after he had really tried to do it on his own. Bobby's school performance improved in two weeks and by the end of that school term he was obtaining average grades.

Another example. A couple, married for seven years, reported not having had sexual intercourse for the last five years due to the husband's worries with his work. In a conjoint session with the couple, the wife was told to start making plans to find herself a lover, just for sexual purposes, without romance or emotional involvement, since both wanted the marriage to last, and since the husband was unable to provide sex due to his worries. The result of this intervention was that he recognized his need for therapy. At the next session they reported that they had enjoyed sex "as newlyweds" twice since they had seen me.

Many exciting examples of paradoxical interventions are found in the authors cited earlier, Erickson (see Haley, 1973) being perhaps the most daring of them all.

Recent Noteworthy Contributions

I will now focus on two of the most outstanding and recent contributions to family hypnotherapy. These are, first, that families use hypnosis and, second, that hypnotic principles and techniques are essential to help families become functional.

Rather than review the works of the many authors who have contributed recently to family hypnotherapy (Calof, 1983; Dammann, 1983; Lankton, 1985; Loriedo, 1985; Mazza, 1983; Ritterman, 1983) or compare them, I want to extract these two main themes regarding the use of hypnosis in family therapy. The above-mentioned authors have discovered effective maneuvers in applying hypnosis to the family group. They have also proposed novel theoretical formulations which have enriched our perception of family interaction. In this respect, for instance, just to reemphasize, Calof (1985) insists on the need to consider both systemic realities and intrapsychic processes; Ritterman (1983) points to masterful hypnotic transactions within the family; the Lanktons (1983) help clarify hypnotic influences through their elegant ecosystemic model of family therapy.

Hypnosis within the family. One of the basic principles regarding hypnotic transactions among family members is enunciated by Ritterman (1983): "We propose that each human being has a capacity for suggestion readiness, an idiosyncratic ability to *turn on* (or off) to a certain type or format of suggestion that can then affect aspects of his psychophysiological functioning" (p. 35). The corollary of this, as it applies to family therapy, follows:

> If an individual is overly suggestible to certain indirect family cues, or unable to turn off to those cues, *the therapist may want to use the trance state to immunize him against such "invisible" directives* . . . (p. 35), (because) the symptomatic state (is) partly a destructive utilization of trance capabilities, in which the symptom-bearer is carrying out some reconciliation of seemingly irreconcilable suggestions from another person or social context, a family context and/or his or her context of mind. (p. 37) (my emphasis)

Thus it is important to become adept at detecting "family hypnosis" in order to transform the hypnotic techniques family members use nonconsciously into therapeutic maneuvers of a counter-inductive nature. To this end, as Ritterman (1983) suggests, the five-step model of the induction process proposed by Erickson and Rossi (1979) is useful and elegant. Assuming that rapport has been established, 1) attention is fixated, via the patient's beliefs and behavior, by focusing attention on inner realities. Then, 2) habitual frameworks and belief systems are depotentiated by means of distraction, shock, surprise, confusion, and dissociation that interrupt the habitual mental processes. This is followed by 3) a subconscious search through indirect hypnotic suggestions, such as implications, questions, or puns. This leads to 4) a subconscious process which activates personal associations and meanings, producing, finally, 5) hypnotic responses, subjectively experienced as autonomous (Erickson & Rossi, 1979, p. 4).

What Ritterman (1983) has pointed out is that "bad hypnosis" is at work in dysfunctional families; the symptom-bearer being hypnotized by the others. This subtle process of family hypnosis appears in many situations. For instance, the father who told the 16-year-old daughter he trusted her with her boyfriend but kept checking on her, either by constant questions or by actually appearing in places where the daughter was, engaged in hypnotic suggestion (the indirect message that "I can't trust you; you'll do something wrong") and, paradoxically, was facilitating her doing something to prove that he couldn't trust her.

Another example is the mother who encouraged her 18-year-old son to talk to her, implying that there was something wrong with him if he did not. But as soon as he would start, she interrupted him, ended his sentences, and reassured him that she knew him better than he knew himself, leading him to clam up and thus finding new reasons to imply again that there was something wrong with him. According to Erickson and Rossi's (1979) five-step model of hypnosis, this mother was challenging his view of himself as being a normal youngster (Step #2) and suggesting that he take a close look at himself to discover that he was not normal (Step #3). Since families share many life events and memories, it is easier for the one using "bad hypnosis" to deepen the trance and produce age regressions and dramatic revivifications by an appeal to many of those past events (Step #4). The result is the hypnotic response which may consist of the son becoming unusually quiet at the mere presence of the mother (Step #5).

The child may also have hypnotic power over the parents. An adopted daughter, 18 years of age, complained that her parents were too old. Her father was 68 and her mother was 62. All her friends' parents were much younger than her own. The child wanted to move in with her cousin whose children were of about the same age as she was. In the hypnotic process, the focus (Step #1) was the age factor which challenged the parents' belief (Step #2) that they were good parents and everything about their parenting was all right. This led to their subconscious search (Step #3) for their motivations in having adopted a child so late in life, as was brought up in many dreams they had since the daughter started this challenge. Both parents had come from emotionally deprived families, a fact that triggered innumerable personal associations in each of them (Step #4). These associations related to feelings of rejection and emotional neglect experienced when growing up. The results (Step #5) were, on the one hand, false attempts on the parents' part to look and act younger and, on the other, a constant spoiling of the daughter, who had become more and more demanding and less and less helpful around the house, while, at the same time, insulting them both privately and publicly. The daughter was ruling the household through her use of "bad hypnosis."

In family treatment, the therapist first learns to observe "family hypnosis" at work and then looks for points of hypnotherapeutic entry, in order to lead the family into inner experiences. The first task, that of observing, is developed through careful self-training. The therapist must *understand the need to develop keen observation skills* in the family therapy session; must *want to practice this observation* at every opportunity that presents itself; and then must do it. There are a few guidelines to sharpen one's awareness and observation of family hypnosis, which are not basically different from the *observation* step in the OLD C model. If hypnosis is right-hemispheric functioning, one looks for manifestations of it, not just in the individual, but either in the individual's talk and behavior or in *the interaction*, usually between two family members. Here, too, one observes the three broad categories of behavior, i.e., figures of speech and language style, important statements, and somatics. It is obvious that the family therapy session, among other things, becomes a living laboratory to observe the interaction between family members. This is one of the great advantages of interviewing a family, as opposed to dealing with only one person at a time.

In the first case mentioned earlier, that of the 16-year-old daughter who complained about her father not trusting her despite his affirmations to the contrary, I observed the father's tender, loving look when addressing the daughter (somatics), and also his use of the word "girl," even in cases where the conversation focused on the young *woman* and her dating. Finally, one or two statements kept appearing in the father's talk which were more emphatic than the rest. These concerned his greater involvement in his daughter's care than other fathers, because of his wife's debilitating illness when his daughter was between seven and 10 years old. The *lead* step of the OLD C model, or the hypnotherapeutic entry, can start at any of these events. I chose the father's loving look by saying: ''I notice how lovingly you look at your daughter. It makes me feel good. (slowing tempo of my speech) Could you slow down and look at her again? (pause) Just like that. (pause) Now, get in touch with your feelings. (at father's slow blinking) Like to let your eyes close? To avoid distractions for a while? (pause) Just fine. (pause) And connect with what you *really* feel about your daughter (pause) at this moment?'' etc. This led the father to admit that in his mind his daughter was still at least five years younger. This, in turn, led to meaningful interactions between daughter and father.

The mother who did not allow her 18-year-old son to communicate verbally with her, even though she constantly asked him to do so, was given the task to express more and more, during the therapy session, what she thought was on her son's mind. This aspect of their interaction made her ''hypnotic power'' over him so weak that after a couple of sessions their verbal communication had become meaningful to them, respectful, and mature. Only then was this family able to work on becoming more functional. In their interaction there were also many somatic cues and important statements. However, the clinical choice of the point of entry depends on many factors. I chose the aspect of her language style with her son because I was more aware of it than of other elements in their interaction (a subjective factor always present), and because that was one of the main symptoms which left the father uninvolved. My choice was also influenced by my desire to test whether this was truthfully a real therapeutic issue, which it turned out to be. If it had not worked, I would have used any of the three main hypnotic categories (somatics, language style, important statements) which can be used to lead the clients into a new experience of their communication.

Finally, the 18-year-old and her parents, were invited "to get inside" of themselves and check their feelings when the daughter, nonconsciously, changed her facial expression (somatics) to one of anger, while stating that she wanted to move away from her home. This elicited the information about the parents' emotionally deprived childhood which had not been communicated to the daughter before. Because of this new awareness of her parents' feelings, the daughter was able to change her perception or mind-set, which resulted in the parents' age issue becoming less important and that of her self-worth and her adoption being dealt with effectively.

The New Hypnosis, as the above discussion indicates, lends itself very well to developing the skill of using "family hypnosis" therapeutically. What the family has been doing ineffectively and counterproductively can be turned around for their benefit. The awareness of this aspect of family communication we owe to Ritterman (1983), whose "dialectical" approach to family therapy is a welcome relief from the rigid systemic approach elevated recently to the status of religious dogma in many family therapy circles. By "dialectical" she means a therapeutic intervention which integrates both the family system within its own culture and the interior level of the individual's frame of mind. To focus on one side of the dialectic at the expense of the other impoverishes our intervention and effectiveness.

The need for family hypnotherapy. The unproven dogma that insight is essential for change was successfully challenged by Erickson (Haley, 1973; Erickson & Rossi, 1979). The brief therapy model developed by the Mental Research Institute is an excellent example of how to help people change by activating right-hemispheric mental processes. The application of hypnotic principles to family therapy (what Watzlawick [1983] calls "hypnosis without trance") consists of *helping individuals alter their mental frame of reference* by encouraging them to try new ways of behaving. This getting outside the frame of reference in which they have been imprisoned gives people a new existential freedom to be different. This was the mastery of Erickson. When people are able to behave in ways they either had not considered possible for themselves or had made into strict prohibitions, they change their immediate behavior (the symptomatic reason for seeking therapy). But they also change their self-perception and definition of their own world. A real inner transformation takes place. On the other hand, when the answer to the question Why? is assumed to be essential for change, people are kept in their habitual way of perceiving themselves and their world. Their "reality," which is the ultimate reason for their problem, remains unchanged.

The New Hypnosis starts from the datum of experience, that reality is a perceptual phenomenon, therefore, it is subjective. This is what epistemology calls *second-order reality*, the only reality we deal with in therapy generally, and especially in family therapy. Consequently, if family therapy is to be effective, it must be hypnotic because one's reality or world image, or one's mental frame of reference, is not changed by argument and reasons but only by one's different inner experience. To sum up this important point, Watzlawick's (1978) words are helpful:

> If (*what* has to change is one's reality or world image, and *how* to change it depends on language, this) reveals the inappropriateness of a procedure which essentially consists of translating this analogic language into the digital language of explanation, argument, analysis, confrontation, interpretation and so forth, and which, through this translation, repeats the mistake which made the sufferer seek help in the first place—instead of learning the patient's right-hemispheric language and utilizing it as the royal road to therapeutic change. (pp. 46–47)

In family therapy we find people fixated in their frames of reference regarding their relationships, their values, their expectations, and so on. This refers to both intrapsychic and interpersonal processes. Each individual perceives the situation differently, although, as members of the same family, they also have "shared perceptions." Besides the intrapsychic, they also relate according to a family structure which is seldom questioned or challenged by them, but which affects their world image.

I consider the hypnotic approach *essential* to family therapy, because the effectiveness of this approach hinges on dealing with these two processes simultaneously, and hypnosis is the best method to reach both the intrapsychic and interpersonal conjointly. IT is interesting, as Calof (1985) points out, that family therapists, such as Whitaker, have realized that entry points for family therapy are found when patients show hypnotic-like behavior. Rather than wait for these occurrences, the family hypnotherapist can facilitate these entry points. One of the great advantages of working hypnotically (avoiding left-hemispheric activation and fostering experiential thinking) is to generate affective intensity, to get people in touch with what they are actually feeling. As Calof (1985) explains, one can give assignments such as visiting one's parents, if intergenerational dynamics are sought, by adding hypnotic suggestions which will regulate the affect to be experienced in such tasks. In the session itself, for instance, hypnosis makes it possible for one spouse to be in touch with other aspects of the self or of the partner. It allows them to actually ''see'' other aspects, faces, ages, which might be at work at the time but which would be ignored if the therapeutic work would continue in a left-hemispheric fashion.

Another advantage of hypnosis, also according to Calof (1985), is the increase of intimacy. This can be accomplished by sharing the trance in the session, using mutual hypnosis (Araoz, 1978), or by inducing a ''dream'' about something specific in the session, or suggesting that family members have a dream at night related to the issue they are working on. Hypnotic suggestions can also release restricted or unexpressed feelings between a couple or between children and parents. Another aspect of hypnotic work is that it can produce a quick increase of loyalty among family members or transfer loyalty from parents to spouse.

These suggestions, coming from the couple's desire to improve or enrich their relationship, are given through a variety of techniques (many of which are also used in Traditional Hypnosis), such as age progression, so that they experience themselves after many years together and looking back on the problems they had when they were in family therapy. This technique can be very powerful with children, especially teenagers. Other methods available to the family hypnotherapist are shared fantasies, projections into the future, resolution of past hurts and painful experiences, and so forth. The hypnotic experience may be used with one family member alone, or with two who may be working on a particular issue, or with the whole family at once.

To illustrate these current family hypnotherapy techniques, three case vignettes follow. There was a childless couple who wanted to conceive but were unable to do so. Finally, in their mid-thirties, they adopted a boy. By the time the family came to therapy, the son was 15 and involved in drug use. The turning point in the therapy came when both parents, in hypnosis during the family session, relived their discussions and decision made 15 years earlier to adopt a child. In trance they talked about their fears, hopes, love, and so forth. Their son was so moved by this experience that he was invited to move hypnotically into the future and meet his parents when they were in their sixties. The parents joined in the trance. Great affect was experienced and without any further suggestions the family situation improved dramatically and quickly.

In a similar case, another family (the father black, the mother white, with two black sons born from the marriage) came to family therapy because the father was in love with the wife's divorced sister. The sister was encouraging the affair and refused to join the family for therapy, although everybody (mother and children) knew about the situation. Though in love, the father was ambivalent about leaving his family. Through age regression, the couple was able to relive their own love affair, the difficulties encountered due to the interracial issue, their feelings at the birth of their two children, etc. Again, through age progression, they "attended" their children's college graduations and their children's marriages. "In the future," they looked back at the current difficulty. The outcome was that the husband discovered personality traits and features in his sister-in-law which he perceived as negative and aversive. The extramarital love affair then ended.

A third family complained about fighting between the parents, loss of sexual interest, and fear that the seven-year-old daughter might be negatively affected by the atmosphere of animosity in the household. In this case, an expansion of the dyadic context through hypnotic suggestion and cuing was effected. Both spouses had current and longstanding communication problems with their parents. As an operative hypothesis it was decided that both were using the other as a target of the frustration with their other sex parent. In hypnosis, they learned "to see" the other sex parent each time they felt irritation with the spouse. This technique alone diminished the antagonism and they were able to concentrate on other aspects of their relationship which the constant fighting was not allowing to emerge.

Some family hypnotherapists find that their approach facilitates the involvement of resistant family members by hypnotically inviting other family members to review good memories associated with the reluctant party or by verbalizing positive feelings about that family member.

Activation of personality parts through hypnosis can help families accept more constructively behaviors which are otherwise intolerable. In one session, a father said, referring to his 16-year-old son, "I'm so afraid he's going to turn out like me. It took me years to overcome my tendency to lie. Now I see the same trait in him." This suggested the activation of his insecure personality side. By eliciting it hypnotically, the son was encouraged to activate his "mature" part and to let that part respond to his father. This exchange became greatly reassuring to the father and strengthened the son to become the mature self he had inside of him.

Mental rehearsal of difficult family events, such as a child leaving home, hospitalization of a family member, and even the death of a spouse or child is another example of the value of applying hypnotic techniques in family therapy.

In addition, a couple can be taught to use self-hypnosis, individually or mutually, in order to facilitate communication of feelings and of one's inner life. This approach is useful in practically any aspect of the couple's interaction. In the sexual area, as I have indicated elsewhere (Araoz and Bleck, 1982) hypnosis can free the couple to express themselves more spontaneously and to enrich their sexual encounters.

MY APPROACH IN FAMILY HYPNOTHERAPY

I start from the theoretical position that the family system is made up of and affects the inner perceptions of the individual members. The inner processes are at work, independently of the system as well as in the system. Because of this, I am very interested in any manifestations of negative self-hypnosis (Araoz, 1981, 1982a) and how it may affect members of the family. To uncover negative self-hypnosis I may ask, "What comes to mind when you think of the current problem in the family?" Rather than encourage immediate verbalization, I suggest that they stay with what is going on inside and experience it fully. Only later do we talk, following the OLD C model outlined in Chapter 4. At this point we compare notes among family members. Then I ask them to think of the family *without the current problem*—as it can be ideally. Once more I encourage them to get into that mental picture as fully as possible, paying attention to every single detail. After they have had some time to get involved in their inner realities, they exchange impressions and discuss what can realistically be expected. From here on, I use any and all of the techniques mentioned in previous sections of this chapter.

I find that hypnotic methods work effectively in all cases, except when there is thought disturbance and difficulty to "get out of imagery." In all other cases, the OLD C model helps to find points of hypnotherapeutic entry at almost every moment. Assuming that people are always dealing with imprints, introjects, and projections, it is easy to identify these inner experiences by inviting them "to stay with what's going on inside" and by encouraging them to intensify their inner experiences. This becomes the best naturalistic induction in itself.

To summarize, I find several situations in which family therapy becomes more effective by means of hypnotic techniques. The following categories are given as a partial list of situations. It is not intended to be an exhaustive list.

Insight Without Change

The OLD C approach in family therapy is extremely helpful with families in which one or more members have experience of individual or couple therapy. Such people have been conditioned *to talk*, as if therapy's effectiveness (the process of human transformation) were in direct proportion to the amount of verbalization, understanding, and intellectualization. These families, usually "guided" by very articulate parents, are ready to describe in detail the great insights they have about their problems. In order to stop them gently but firmly, I make it clear that "my therapy is very different from other approaches. Inner experience is paramount; talk is secondary." I then add immediately, "Right now go inside of yourself and check your reaction to my words." I give them time to get in touch with their inner reactions. If they start talking, I ask them not to speak but to "wait and first become fully aware of what's going on inside." Initially, it is difficult to recondition them, but with perseverance the results *are* rewarding.

A family was referred by a pediatrician because the 12-year-old daughter, Robin, an only child, had been found with marijuana and had admitted to smoking it regularly. The parents, both professionals, spent very little time with Robin, even on weekends. Both had been in individual psychotherapy for several years. They made valiant efforts to let me know their mistakes in rearing Robin; chief among them was that both used marijuana regularly. But even though they had talked to Robin and had attempted to improve the family situation, including reducing the use of "pot," she was not cooperative. I asked Robin to try to remember how she felt when smoking marijuana and encouraged her to relive the experience. She was able to do this and her parents became curious about it. In trance, Robin expressed how "pot" made her feel less lonely, more secure about herself, and less angry at her parents. We identified the exact moment when she wanted to smoke and what she expected would happen when she did. This was the beginning of a new relationship between parents and daughter. She agreed to use her "thought of pot" to go to her parents and feel better by dealing with them. After three weeks she had not used marijuana and the parents had enjoyed new "fun things" with Robin, such as taking her to an amusement park, going sailing with her, and attending a concert together. After three months, nobody in the family was using marijuana and the family situation was much improved.

No Awareness of Each Other's Feelings

Many parents fall into the trap of believing that they know their children thoroughly and that they can read their children's minds. This was the case of the Y family. The presenting problem was constant fighting among the three children (Al, 14; Beth and Carl, 13). The fighting made the parents ostensibly angry. During the first session, I suggested that the children "get into their parents' heads," encouraging them to get in touch with what they thought their parents were thinking about the three children, without telling each other what was going on in their own minds. After a brief moment of silence, I suggested that they write down these thoughts. Then, with the aid of their notes, we had a round table discussion. Al said: "They wish they had never had us. They feel they have failed with us." Beth put it this way: "They are sorry we are part of the family." Carl read his notes: "They hate us. I feel they don't want to bother with us. They only want to show us off: We should be good and nice. Then they can forget about us." This came as a shock to the parents. Even the three children were surprised about their general agreement. The parents admitted their ambivalence about their children. In front of them, during subsequent sessions, both parents got in touch with different personality parts, the one who complained about the children and the one who wanted to be the perfect parent. The children reacted positively to this truthful admission of ambivalence on the part of the parents and, at my suggestion, tried "to help" their parents accept their ambivalence. Immediately an improvement in the family atmosphere was noticed. This continued in the following weeks when children and parents were able to enter into "contracts" to satisfy more fully each others' needs.

To have taken a less experiential approach in this case probably would have delayed the therapy and kept the real problem hidden much longer.

Adult-Child Dichotomy

The notorious "generation gap" often occurs because of a lapse in memory. In many conflicts between parents and their offspring, hypnotic techniques help them to become more aware and sensitive of each other. Using time distortion, for instance, parents are invited to go back and relive times when they were the child's age, while the child is asked to project herself into the future when she is a parent. In the New Hypnosis this time-honored hypnotic technique is introduced without any formal induction, almost in a playful manner. However, once people start making the effort to move chronologically back or forth in their mind, the technique is taken very seriously.

A family arrived with the following problem. The daughter, 23, a computer expert living in her own apartment, had been offered a wonderful opportunity for professional advancement in a remote part of the country. The parents, now in their early seventies and in excellent health, insisted that she had the responsibility of staying near them in case "something happens to one of us." Reasons and argument pro and con would have led nowhere. Hypnotically the parents were able to confront their fears of sickness and death, while reliving their youthful years when they did what was good for them. The daughter, who had requested the family therapy sessions, was able to recognize her parents' fears and together they made provisions for emergencies and future visits. She felt free to move without guilt; the parents recognized their daughter's right to live her life without the burden of responsibility for their welfare. A relationship that had been dominated by resentment and bitterness became loving, car-ing, and mutually giving. Hypnosis was also used to help the parents ''see'' their daughter in the future, accomplished in her career and happy which was, indeed, what they wanted for her.

Plateaus

Often in family therapy, as in any other form of therapy, it appears that no progress is being made. In these cases, to employ the OLD C model with the whole family, produces a meaningful change of pace. Following is an example of this maneuver. Joe, a military officer, Nancy, his wife, their 18-year-old daughter, and their 15-year-old son had requested therapy because Nancy felt helpless with the children. The son, Bobby, was getting drunk too often and the daughter, Lisa, was ''acting as a prostitute,'' while Joe was mostly absent from home and generally disinterested, pursuing his military advancements. The family had become more cohesive and cooperative after four sessions of therapy. Lisa, far from being sexually promiscuous (her mother's fear), had kept to a reasonable curfew, and Bobby had stopped drinking beer to excess when Joe became more involved with him. Nancy had recognized her sexual frustration, projected onto her daughter, and the couple had become more aware of each other's needs, allowing for more time with each other and more satisfying sexual activity. Much of this change had been accomplished through the techniques mentioned in this chapter.

At this point in therapy (fifth session) the changes obtained were too fresh for the family to feel comfortable with them. At the same time, everything was proceeding smoothly but there was a feeling of impasse in the therapy session. I asked the family to relax and to allow themselves to have some form of a dream of their family functioning happily and without problems. Each one was encouraged ''to get into'' his or her own dream for a while, before discussing it together. Joe reported a situation where his wife and he were playing tennis, enjoying the game. After the game they were relaxing over a cool refreshment, holding hands and talking leisurely about their forthcoming vacation without the children, "a new honeymoon." Nancy's dream was of a party where her husband was attentive to her, making her feel loved and important. Lisa saw herself shopping with her mother and feeling very happy talking to her about a young man she was interested in. Bobby had "dreamt" about him and his father going on a hike through the woods in the area, birdwatching and talking. I asked them first to try to understand these dreams as real possibilities which they could now plan to execute and, second, to become aware of the fact that all four dreams expressed feelings of comfort and peace with each other. Then I invited them to plan during the session when and how they could make their dreams come true. The family therapy session became very active and involving for all of them. The family situation continued to improve from this session on and therapy was ended after two more sessions.

Fights and Blaming

The family therapy session should never be allowed to become the site of in-family fighting, accusations, and indictments. However, many families are so used to arguments that it becomes possible for them to end up screaming at each other during the session, unless the family therapist has effective interventions to redirect their interaction. The New Hypnosis, being naturalistic and not formalized, lends itself to intervene effectively in these cases. The therapist observes keenly every alteration of mood in her clients, according to the OLD C model. The moment the expressions of anger tend to become unproductive through blaming and accusations, it is useful to invite the family member experiencing the anger to "go inside of yourself" and get in touch with all the affect that is being felt. The family member is encouraged to experience in his or her imagination all the anger, to become aware of any images that are elicited, to follow them and experience them fully, as well as any associations to earlier scenes originated spontaneously, without talking about his or her inner awareness. After a while, the discussion centers only on those inner experiences. Frequently, very meaningful material comes to consciousness, helping the whole family understand better and handle more effectively the anger that previously had gone out of control.

A couple who had been separated for over a year after 12 years of marriage sought family therapy because of the school truancy of their 17-year-old son. Both parents were afraid of his anger manifested in outbursts of rage and violence, such as smashing furniture (though he had never attacked either of his parents). Several times during the family therapy sessions, the son showed signs of such anger. He was told to proceed as indicated above—to get in touch with what he was feeling inside. What emerged was the anger experienced, but not expressed, towards his mother when he was 10 and his father had left the household (during the couple's first separation). At that age, he had blamed the mother, believing his father had left them because she was "mean to Dad." In the family therapy sessions, they were able to help each other understand these events which had taken place seven years before but had never been discussed.

To have allowed a free expression of anger would have been wasteful of time at best, and destructive of family communication at worst. By using this hypnotic approach, the anger became constructive and helpful to the family communication. The son's truancy problem disappeared without directly focusing on it. I see most expression of anger as a surface affect. Not much is gained in terms of inner awareness by giving it free rein. Only by going below the surface can a person become aware of where the anger comes from and how it is ignited. Hypnosis provides a quick technique to truly get in touch with the whole, deep reality of one's anger.

These then are a few situations in working with families where the hypnotic approach makes the therapist's interventions more effective in a short period of time. The OLD C model, modified to fit the setting in which several people are involved, is convenient, elegant, and effective to help the family change constructively.

CONCLUSION

The New Hypnosis lends itself very easily to family therapy. The chapter has reviewed many approaches within the hypnotic model, all of which have one element in common: awareness of inner realities facilitates the workings of the family system. Awareness is not understanding. The latter, in my view, is an intellectual making sense of something going on within the family. The former is an acknowledgment, an owning of some psychological realities either ignored or denied previously. Since awareness expands one's perception and, consequently, one's choices, by increasing or expanding awareness families view themselves differently and, in so doing, they discover new possibilities, new options, for their interaction.

7

Our Inner
Healer

This chapter is the natural extension of my Negative Self-Hypnosis (NSH) concept to the area of physical health. Since there is considerable current enthusiasm about eniatric healing (*en* = within; *iatros* = healer, physician), which I share, I thought it beneficial to present an overview of this vast and complex area of interest. The New Hypnosis, because of its naturalness, is especially useful to activate "our inner healer." Eniatric healing takes place every second of our lives. Unlike machines, our body is constantly repairing itself, healing itself. We would not survive without our inner healer constantly at work. When the New Hypnosis is applied to physical health, it activates this miraculous process of self-healing. In harmony with the principles of the New Hypnosis, I emphasize throughout this chapter health over sickness, health-maintenance techniques over methods to recover from sickness, and a general attitude of trust in our inner healer, rather than a preoccupation with disease.

Although traditional Western medicine had lost its soul and had become overly mechanized (Illich, 1976), we are now witnessing a hopeful turn which views the *sick person* with greater interest than the abstract sickness itself, as the new emphasis on holistic medicine shows. Regardless of its faults and imperfections, holistic medicine is welcome. In this respect—focusing on

119

the individual and the natural healing forces of the human body—
the New Hypnosis can be of special benefit to both laymen and
professionals.

The medical community does not seem to be ready to give up
the reality it has invented, as Watzlawick (1984) would put it,
when it comes to admitting that psyche affects soma (Illich, 1976).
As a group, medicine accepts the Cartesian dichotomy of mind
and body, being reluctant to admit the powerful effects of mind
on body, pointing to a more unified somatopsychic reality. In the
last few years, with the development of the science of psychoneuroimmunology (see Ader, 1981), evidence has been mounting
regarding the effect of "thoughts" on the functioning of the
body. As Pelletier (1979) said, when it comes to physical health,
the mind can be a healer or a slayer. But the medical community
has often reacted with hostility or indifference to this possibility
(Polanyi, 1964). An example of the reluctance to even look at this
fascinating area is what happened to one of my articles published
in the *Journal of Psychosocial Oncology* (Araoz, 1984a). The fourth
part of that article, which dealt with "hypnosis to activate the natural healing process," was not published. What I wrote follows.

Mears (1979), an Australian physician who has written important material on hypnosis, uttered the unspeakable in many medical circles: "We should be prepared to face inevitable criticism
and take the big step of attempting to influence cancer growth
by psychological means" (p. 978). He has reported a number of
cases of regression of cancer following intensive meditation, a
hypnotic method he devised. The field of psychoneuroimmunology is only in its infancy, but the evidence is accumulating in
the direction of a linkage between the healing mechanisms and
mental activity, particularly hypnosis. Hall's (1983) review of the
effect of hypnosis on the functioning of the immune system,
strengthened by his own research on T and B cell immunity function, led him to conclude that we may be on our way to influenc-
ing physical diseases with cognitive and psychological processes,
since a number of illnesses result from either an underreaction
or an overreaction of the immune system.

It is generally accepted today that psychosocial factors can and often do contribute to a physical disease. The use of hypnosis to potentially modify immune function in order to alter the biochemical factors responsible for many physical diseases results from a pragmatic outlook. It seems to state that if it certainly does not harm the patient (Coe and Ryken, 1979) and if it may, at least in some cases, produce positive results (Hall, 1983), hypnosis should be tried as an integral part of the treatment. None of the reports and studies reviewed by Hall (1983) or by Finkelstein and Howard (1983) use hypnosis exclusively to cure cancer; accepted medical treatment is applied simultaneously or concomitantly.

The hypnotic suggestions given while the patient is encouraged to relax and use positive imagery center around the reality of the healing forces operating in the body. The focus is on this reality rather than on the negative effects of the disease. The patient is asked before hypnosis to describe how she imagines these health forces at work in her body. Let us assume that the patient says she sees them as waves of different colors emanating from her brain. In this case, the hypnotherapist may suggest that she connect these waves with her breathing and that she try to make them more intense with every breath:

> Without forcing your breathing, just imagine those waves of health in your body following the rhythm of your breathing. Check if you notice anything else in these waves of health, active in your body. Is there any change in their color? Any sound or music? How far do they reach inside of your body? Are they slowly, but very effectively, reaching the area in your body that needs them the most? Keep thinking about this wonderful reality in your body, while you breathe and say to yourself: ''The health forces in me can become stronger and stronger. I want to enjoy this thought and come back to it many times after hypnosis. I want to think more and more about the health waves in me; many times during the day . . . the health forces in me becoming stronger with the medical treatment. The health forces in me doing their job of healing my body with the help of the

therapy. The health forces . . . part of me, growing, stronger with every breath I take.''

If the patient does not have any mental image of her health
forces, just the gentle repetition of suggestions similar to those
described above, while in a state of relaxation, is encouraged. I
have found that these patients progressively start to associate
the kinetic experience of relaxation with the healing suggestions.
Thus, as was mentioned before, imagery takes the form of a kinetic experience rather than that of a mental picture. However,
from that kinetic experience, often memories of relaxing places
start to shape up in their minds and some visualization takes
place.

It should be noted that the hypnotic suggestions are not built
on medical science or careful anatomical or physiological descriptions. All these are usually left-hemispheric activities: a logical,
rational way of thinking. Rather, in hypnosis the experiential way
of thinking is activated: right-hemispheric, primary processes.
Through these, what patients *imagine, feel, or sense* about the life
forces in them is utilized for the hypnotic experience.

There is some evidence to believe that hypnosis can aid in the
prevention of cancer (Finkelstein and Howard, 1983). A three-
year pilot study with 43 persons considered to be at high risk for
cancer produced encouraging results, especially because the method used was so simple: a 10-minute audio cassette was played
by the subjects at least four times a week for three years. Data
were collected after both one year and three years. The taped
audio message included a relaxation induction, suggestions for
higher self-esteem, contra-cancer suggestions, and a final session
to deepen the hypnotic experience.

It has been demonstrated that humans are frequently, if not
constantly, engaged in some form of self-talk (see T. X. Barber,
1979a). To alter the content of this flow results in mood change
(Araoz, 1981). Mood and psychological states have a definite effect on the progress of disease (see Schleifer, Keller, McKegney,
and Stein, 1980; Shekelle, Raynor, Ostfeld, Garron, Bieliauskas,
Liu, Maliza & Oglesby, 1981). The conclusion from these facts
is that a method which helps people in these processes may have

a beneficial impact on the progress of disease. This method is hypnosis, and even though we are still ignorant of many of its aspects, the advisability of proceeding with further research in this area stands to reason.

The above concepts would be considered rather commonplace among psychosomatic specialists (see, e.g., Weinstock, 1984). Rather than referring to the mind affecting the body (two entities of different natures interacting), we could think in terms of information processing (Bowers, 1977). What is the process by which semantic input is decoded as somatic output? In Bowers and Kelly's (1979) words: "If we presuppose that the mind and the body are *linked by informational processes*, instead of being separated by a philosophical abyss, the facts of hypnotic healing may be regarded more as *a way of accessing these processes*, than as an affront to the time-honored gap between two separate realms" (p. 502) (my emphasis).

HYPNOTIC PRINCIPLES AT WORK

The consequences of the above are important. To begin with, the statements a doctor makes or the words used in referring to cancer (or to any other disease for that matter) and to its medical treatment can act as powerful hypnotic suggestions which may affect the course of the disease: Semantic input decoded as somatic output. Indeed, in the medical approach to disease one finds roughly two main trends: that which focuses *on the disease itself* or the afflicted organs, disregarding the semantic input, and that which regards *the person* suffering from the disease and being careful about the words (suggestions) which may start the psychosomatic process. Kleinman and his collaborators (1978) pointed out that American physicians tend to treat the "disease," often ignoring the "illness," i.e., the personal experience of the disease and the idiosyncratic meaning it has for the patient. Remen (1980) referred to the suffering that stems from the personal meaning and interpretation of any disease. Is the person really cured when her inner realities connected with the disease are ignored? Can we continue to view mind and body as separate and independent of each other? The evidence, carefully reviewed by T. X. Barber (1981b; 1984a), forces us to answer no unequivocally to both questions.

At the core of the mind-body interaction we find suggestions, namely, meanings or ideas imbedded in words which are spoken by one person and deeply accepted by another (T. X. Barber, 1984a). Suggestions, explicit or not, affect the mind which then affects the body. These suggestions "can be communicated to the cells of the body and to the chemicals within the cells. The cells, then, can change their activities in order to conform to the meanings or ideas which have been transmitted to them" (T. X. Barber, 1984a, p. 116). If these words had not been preceded by more than 40 pages of scientific data, critically presented and evaluated, they would certainly sound like pure nonsense.

It is of historical interest to note that already in the late 19th century the Nancy school had published many detailed cases of diseases affected positively by direct hypnotic suggestions (Bernheim, 1888/1964). They had already accepted the following facts: 1) The human body's nature is to be healthy and well functioning; 2) the human body has powerful resources to maintain its health, to combat pathogens, and to heal itself; 3) the human body will carry out better its healing if nutrition and exercise are monitored and improved; 4) feeling good and positive about oneself benefits the human body; the old-fashioned concept of *happiness* facilitates healing, while negative feelings are obstacles to the inner forces of health; and 5) self-hypnosis is an effective mental tool to generate positive feelings about oneself. My main concern is with #4 and #5, although the first three points are fascinating. (For a review of the evidence concerning those first three facts, see T. X. Barber, 1981b.)

Negative Self-hypnosis

In order fully to understand the fact that good and positive feelings about oneself are beneficial to one's physical body, it is helpful to remember how negative thoughts affect one's health.

This is the reality of negative self-hypnosis (Araoz, 1981) in the physical realm. Lynch (1977), to give one dramatic example, reviewed scientifically the concept of the broken heart and how it may be related to a variety of diseases. The evidence presented cannot be dismissed lightly without violating one's sense of objectivity. The broken heart syndrome is a good example of stress, a perceptual phenomenon, produced not by the event but by one's way of reacting to the event. Stress, on the other hand, consists of negative thoughts, images, memories, and feelings one allows (and therefore, at some point, chooses) under specific circumstances of frustration, disappointment, shattered hopes and dreams, and the like. The literature on stress is extensive and scientifically documented. We know that stress is causatively linked with many diseases, as Selye's (1976) classic studies proved, opening the door to the increasingly growing research in this area (see, e.g., Bowers and Kelly, 1979; Hall, 1983, 1984). The general conclusion is that negative thoughts, images, and feelings are directly related to many diseases and even can lead to death itself, as the studies reported by Engel (1971) indicate.

However, more is known: that specific body functions can be affected and altered by specific beliefs. T. X. Barber (1981b) succinctly reviews the evidence related to several skin diseases, false pregnancy, and size alteration of women's breasts. Hall (1984) gives an overview of the effects of hypnosis on allergic responses, dermatological conditions, the inhibition of the Mantoux Reaction (a tuberculin skin test to detect the presence of tubercule bacilli), and cancer. He concluded: "The literature . . . suggests that *hypnosis may potentially be able to alter immune responses* in order to influence the underlying biochemical factors of physical diseases" (p. 101) (my emphasis). His overly cautious language did not hide completely his positive and optimistic conclusion: Mental processes elicited by words (suggestions) affect biophysiological functioning. If the suggestions produce negative mental processes and are sickness-centered, the disease tends to worsen. If they are positive and health-centered, the body tends to overcome the disease and recover its natural healing strength. In both cases it is semantic input decoded as somatic output.

FOCUS ON HEALTH OR DISEASE?

The New Hypnosis is helpful in shifting our attention from disease to health. Most people in our culture take their health for granted and think of it mostly in negative terms, especially when they are not feeling well. The evidence reviewed by the authors mentioned in this chapter points to the fact that *thinking* about our health forces has good effects on our health. Thinking in this context means, obviously, experiential thinking. Shames and Sterin (1978), taking an eminently pragmatic attitude, advocate New Hypnosis methods for self-healing. They remind us of the great importance of the quality of our mental images in facilitating or inhibiting the natural healing process. However, these authors emphasize what should be a prerequisite or sine qua non condition of any mental activity to promote self-healing. This is the need to examine our holistic reaction to living. Negative feelings, in their explanation, "turn inward and begin to accumulate as toxicity in the system" (p. 90). One must, therefore, deal with these negative feelings and often make decisions to change either one's lifestyle, or values and attitudes, or relationships.

Positive self-hypnosis will be ineffective in self-healing if the person is not correcting abuses which might impede the natural healing process. Common abuses gravitate around diet, poor working habits, and lack of adequate exercise. It is very important to stress with our clients the need to control excessive tobacco smoking or alcohol drinking, as well as awareness of one's general diet so that it becomes well balanced. Working habits comprise a wide variety of behavior, from schedules and vacations to organization and delegation of responsibilities. In the work schedule, the breaks one takes may be as important as the actual time spent working, since the breaks (their quality, length, and frequency) affect the quality of work. Physical exercise, for example, could be fitted in one of the major work interruptions during business hours or reserved for before or after work.

The point to underline is that clients must be made aware of these areas connected with health and should understand the contradiction between positive thoughts and a negative lifestyle.

The sad truth is that negativism, in this case, overpowers positive thoughts. However, once the person respects the laws of nature and exerts control over the three areas mentioned (diet, work-leisure, exercise), self-hypnosis to activate "the Doctor within" becomes a powerful facilitator of health. (The Doctor within is the designation used by Bennett (1981) in a marvellous book which outlines a comprehensive program to keep well.) The truth that imagery and self-hypnosis can become powerful facilitators of health is confirmed by Sheikh, Richardson, and Moleski (1979) in their review of recent experimental evidence. But this truth was also known to the ancients, as Evans-Wentz (1927) reminded us by quoting *The Tibetan Book of the Dead*: "They should have apprehended the method of visualization and applied the illimitable virtue thereof for exhalting one's own condition." This ancient text is far from an exception in "pre-scientific" times. McMahon (1976) investigated beliefs and attitudes in pre-Cartesian thinking, especially regarding imagination. In her words: "The key to an understanding of pre-Cartesian theory lies in recognizing that *imagery was understood to be* as much *a physiological reality* as it is today regarded as a psychological reality" (p. 181) (my emphasis). She also stressed that since imagination had greater powers of control than sensations, anticipation of a feared event was more harmful than the event itself. Because of this, images were deemed to "pervade the body, bind up the heart, clutch at the sinews and vessels, direct the flesh according to its own inclination. Its essence became manifest in its victims' complexion, countenance, posture and gait," (p. 191) as McMahon explains using the poetic expressions of those times. Consistent with this view, much of therapy included imagination.

The change came when the scientific community endorsed Descartes' dualism and separation of mind and body, a development which never contaminated oriental body-mind monism. Eastern medicine considers dualism an illusion (Ikemi and Ikemi, 1983) and, taking advantage of Zen wisdom, subscribes to "taitoku" or bodythinking. That the body and mind are one leads Eastern perception to the principle of sum ergo cogito ("I exist, therefore I think"), the opposite of the Cartesian dictum.

The body is primary, as is shown by the many bodily disciplines developed in Japan, for instance, as a way to self-actualization.

On the other side of this issue is the evidence reported by M'Uzan (1974) regarding the deficiency of imaginary activity in the psychosomatic individual. Such a person, prone to psychogenic disease, seems to find it difficult to fantasize and daydream and is, therefore, less able than others to use imagery in order to activate her natural healing processes (see Sheikh et al., 1979).

To return our attention to hypnosis, it should also be remembered that when the royal commission investigating Mesmer's theory of animal magnetism issued its findings, it vindicated the power of human imagination. The scientists who conducted that inquiry did not question the cures obtained by Mesmer's methods. They attributed them to the imagination of the patients rather than to the existence of animal magnetism.

The next sections will explain the application of New Hypnosis principles and methods in the area of health maintenance and enhancement.

THE NEW HYPNOSIS AND SELF-HEALING

Since the New Hypnosis moves away from ritualized induction and is essentially self-hypnosis (see Chapter 5), it lends itself very well either to activate the health forces in one's body or to energize the healing processes when sickness has upset the normal functioning of the body.

Patients under medical treatment are referred to hypnotherapists either to ameliorate the psychological reactions to the disease, to obtain greater control of their anxiety, to make rest and sleep more effective, or, in general, to improve their whole attitude towards life and health. An adaptation of the OLD C model of the New Hypnosis applies here, too. This process takes five steps:

1) Mental images of disease
2) Mental images of medical treatment
3) Mental images of healing forces at work

4) Mental images of health (2 and 3 combined to overcome 1)
5) Repetition of the above, practiced at home

First, the patient is asked to concentrate on *the mental images related to the disease*. How does the patient imagine what's wrong with her body? The hypnotherapist must give the patient time to capture as many details of the disease-image as possible—size, color, smell, consistency, movement, etc.—and to concentrate on that disease-image until it becomes very vivid. If the patient finds it difficult to discover this mental image, greater relaxation is usually required before returning to the sickness-image. This negative image becomes the focus of attention for a while. The patient must "own" her sickness-image. In the hypnotic experience the patient is encouraged to say to herself such things as, "Yes, this image is inside of me. This image is at work in me. But now that I have uncovered my sickness-image, I can free myself from it. I can let the image go. I can have another image in its place. I can have a health-image, actively working inside of me for my benefit."

The second step is to ask the patient *to imagine the medical treatment* and how this new image modifies the first one or is connected somehow to it. Once more, "slow motion" is the operating principle. The patient must be given plenty of time to allow this image to emerge from the subconscious and to take shape. Once this image has been captured, it is important to let the patient experience it very dynamically, with great energy and movement. I might say, "Notice how strong the medical treatment is, how helpful to your body. It is already changing the sickness in you; it's making it less powerful. The medicine (or whatever medical treatment) is at work now for your benefit; it's helping your inner forces of health to do their job, this very minute." The patient has to arrive at the point where all these suggestions are received in a state of total relaxation, so they become fully accepted. At this stage, I find myself repeating phrases like, "This is the way it is," or "It's perfectly natural for your body to use the strength of the medical treatment," or "It's happening now."

The third step is to request an image of *the internal healing forces*

and energies. Once this appears in consciousness, it is connected
with the two previous images. This is the step where the hypnotherapist must linger. Repetition of the basic concepts in different
forms seems to be of benefit. A sample of suggestions follows:

> Your body is sick, yes, but your body is also healthy. Con-
> nect now with the health energy in your body. Let that health
> energy become very powerful in your experience now. Feel
> it in your brain, feel it in your heart, feel it in your spine,
> feel the health energy everywhere. Say to yourself, ''I want
> to concentrate on the truth of my health forces. I'm alive be-
> cause health energy is flowing through my blood vessels,
> through my nerves, throughout my body. I want to be on
> the side of health.''

As I mentioned in the second step, insistence and patience are
required on the part of the hypnotherapist to make it possible
for patients to change their thinking from a sickness orientation
to a health orientation.

Before proceeding, the clinical case of a 48-year-old male lawyer with progressive rheumatoid arthritis will help elucidate the
process. His sickness-image was a very sticky, glue-like material,
alive and growing around his joints and muscles, especially in
his arms where the pain had been most severe. The medication
he was taking at the time appeared in his mental screen as a powerful fluid that stopped the growth of the sickness. The health
forces were then visualized as an electric current, activated by
the powerful medication fluid, and not only stopping the growth
of the disease but actually reducing the size of the sticky, glue-
like material. The end result, after three hypnotic sessions, was
a harmonious interaction which produced his health-image, a
powerful and radiant force, flowing to the sound of military
marches and revitalizing his whole being.

These three steps constitute the first part of the healing process. The next step is *the enhancement of step three combined with
step two,* finding the imaginary area of the body in which the healing forces start (for most people either the brain or the heart) and
intensifying that mental image with as many sensory details as

possible. The images of the medical treatment at work and those of the health energy using the medical treatment are now combined to make an impact on the sickness-image. Time must be taken to experience progressively how the health forces, with the help of the medical treatment, are affecting the disease; how they are reducing it, weakening it, or destroying it. In many cases the patient visualizes the disease as very strong, active, and alive. In these instances time must be spent in imagining the fight between health and disease. The patient should be encouraged "to pretend" that the health forces win and overcome the sickness. In this connection it should be noted that the inability to enter into this positive imagery may indicate the presence of a death wish. The activation of personality parts (see Chapter 3) is a useful technique to identify the presence of such self-defeating forces and to work through them.

This fourth step, then, is what Jaffe (1980) calls *the healing images*. Patients are helped to recognize and own their specific healing image. In the case just mentioned, the patient visualized the electric current as coming from his heart, having a pleasant silvery color and becoming brighter with each heart beat, "much like a digital clock, like pulsing," as he put it. He was encouraged to feel the healing current of light traveling all over his body and then, slowly, concentrating especially on his arms. Once this was experienced, the healing electric current continued its work with its energizing music, using the powerful fluid (the medication) to become brighter, stronger, and more effective, sharpening its focus on the right elbow and then on the left elbow, on the right shoulder and then on the left, and so on.

The final step is unhurried *repetition at home* of the previously described four steps. To make this more effective, I encourage patients to keep a written record of their daily practice.

The New Hypnosis makes this healing process more natural than when elaborate inductions are used. The patient is introduced to the Doctor within by pointing to the images that spontaneously come to his awareness when he "thinks" about his sickness. Once step one is taken in this almost casual manner, it is easy to proceed through the next three steps, ending with the recommendation to practice repeatedly this mind exercise in private. In the case of the patient mentioned earlier, the doctors were surprised at the rapid improvement he experienced. In three months after he started practicing self-hypnosis, the pain was gone, his freedom of movement had improved 70% in his estimation, and he had returned to the normal activities of a busy professional life.

AN ATTITUDE OF HEALTH

The benign view of one's subconscious mind (Erickson and Rossi, 1979) is a characteristic of the nonpsychoanalytical view advocated by the followers of Erickson. If hypnosis is a natural, healthy activity of the mind, that part of our nervous system responsible for the experience of hypnosis is considered to be positive. From this view, it is not difficult to extend the beneficial influence of the subconscious mind to physical well-being, especially if we move away from Cartesian dualism. Mind and body are one, and the subconscious is seen as the part of us that is responsible for our health and well-being, whether this manifests itself physically, mentally, spiritually, emotionally, or in a combination of these modalities of our being.

I should add here that Erickson's insistence on the benign nature of the subconscious mind is not a naive belief in the goodness of humans. As I understand it, the subconscious mind refers to the activities of the subcortical brain. By its essence, the subconscious is a positive force, "responsible" for the optimal functioning of our being. This includes our physical self—all the complicated changes that take place every second of our existence in every cell of our bodies. And it also includes our nonphysical self—feelings, emotions, and other cognitions (or mentations, as the early psychologists called them).

By nature, then, the function of the subconscious is to keep us alive, healthy, and happy. However, as we can damage our bodily organs through many abuses, personally and culturally inflicted on the body, so too can we impede the benign functioning of our subconscious through emotional abuses. These emotional abuses are erroneous beliefs, false values, toxic attitudes and the like, which we have been ingesting since infancy. By the time we are adults most of us have a subconscious that has been damaged and whose originally benign function has been stifled by all those emotional abuses.

The appeal to the benign subconscious is an attempt *to restore* its positive and good influence rather than to assume that it is intact. What most forms of therapy attempt to do is to purify the subconscious so that the person can benefit from its original benign function; hence, they start by removing the emotional toxicity (neurosis, negative scripts, irrational beliefs, or whatever term is used by different schools of psychotherapy).

My New Hypnosis method assumes the benign *nature* of the subconscious and attempts to restore it to its original function. For instance, the concern with negative self-hypnosis, especially at the beginning of treatment, responds to this notion of purifying the subconscious from emotional toxicity before effective goals are reached. Metanoia (or inner transformation) is possible only after the purification of the subconscious.

Consequently, the attitude of health is fostered by both the view of hypnosis as natural and the understanding of the subconscious as a positive and beneficial force within us. Hence, many clients can be helped to have a more effective view of themselves by emphasizing health more than sickness. People who are overly concerned about disease, or who worry about minor physical symptoms, people who don't take good care of their bodies, and those who take their health for granted can all be taught to remember more often the reality of their health energy.

The following is a brief sequence of suggestions related to health following the five steps mentioned above which assume that the person has spent a moment in the process of entering the alternate state of mind called hypnosis. At that point, the therapist may continue:

> Now that you are relaxed, notice your smooth breathing. Your body has found its own comfortable rhythm of breathing. It's possible for you to enjoy it even more. Every breath can be enjoyed. Think of your breathing in connection with

your health energy. Imagine your health energies becoming stronger, more active with every breath. You may become curious about your health energy. How does it appear in your mind? (Give the person a chance to respond.) What sort of force is this, flowing throughout your body? Now at work in every part of you. A lot of movement and activity in your finger tips, for instance? Great activity and movement in your earlobes? Are you getting into it? And your health forces are there, now, energizing, revitalizing, supervising, healing. Do you feel them? And while you breathe, peaceful- ly, comfortably, your health energy continues to flow, like a mighty power. Fix your attention on it. How does your en- ergy appear in your mind? (According to the response, con- tinue.) See it even more clearly. Experience it fully. Any col- or? Any sound or music? Any temperature change in your body? Where? Enjoy every sensation. Your health energy is you. A part of you you don't think about often. It's the do- main of your inner mind. Allow this energy to radiate in ev- ery one of the trillions of cells in your body. In your heart, in your liver, in your lungs, in your kidneys, in your pan- creas, in your stomach, in your intestines, in every internal organ, in every part of you. Let the force radiate, shine, en- ergize, purify, heal. Let the force go to your brain and radi- ate through your spine, along the nerve cells throughout the body, carried by the nerve impulses and carried by the blood, rejuvenating every organ, every part of you. See yourself surrounded by this energy of life and of health as if your whole body were radiating, fully alive, shining. Enjoy this energy which is you.

These suggestions may give the experienced hypnotherapist sufficient ideas to construct her own sequence for the benefit of her clients. When she uses this method, it is useful to devise, with the client's cooperation, a phrase or message-to-self similar to Cue's famous ''Every day in every way I'm getting better and better,'' to be repeated as often as possible during the day, while going about one's daily business. In connection with the above practice, such a phrase or message can become a post-hypnotic signal to reactivate the experience had in the hypnotic practice.

It is useful to connect such a health message with some circumstance of daily living. In metropolitan areas, a simple relationship could be established with the traffic lights, so that whenever the patient sees a green light or go sign, she reactivates the "go" of her health forces. On the other hand, the red or stop sign may be associated with relaxing, stopping to take care of oneself or stopping one's neglect of the body. Whatever the connection is, it is essential to establish a means of reminding oneself of one's intent to activate the health energy in oneself. Only one of these associations should be suggested. It should not be changed until the client has succeeded in establishing it and experiencing it spontaneously and without thinking.

The attitude of health, then, is very much in accord with the New Hypnosis' positive and constructive view of the mind. It can be a helpful antidote against the sickness orientation fostered by manufacturers of medicinal products and by the medical establishment (see Illich, 1976). This health attitude goes along with the natural tendency of all living matter to attain integration, to be at its best, and to express itself fully, as Nobel Prize winner Szent-Gyoergyi (1974) proved.

This attitude of health extends to times when we are not well. Then, we must use medical means such as consulting a physician or healer or taking medication. But when we don't feel well, although we know our sickness is not such that it requires medical intervention, the method described in this section can transform our sickness into personal growth and self-learning. Jaffe (1980) proposes "that illness is an occasion to begin a positive transformation . . . an opportunity to being an exploration of the self and an expansion of inner knowledge" (pp. 231–232). His view that illness expresses a lack of integration in the ill person lends itself to New Hypnosis methods. As a matter of fact, his dialogue between the conscious and subconscious selves "to share information and work toward the mutual goal of fulfilling the inner person" (Jaffe, 1980, p. 232) is a marvelous application of the New Hypnosis. Experiencing the pain or sickness as an expression of the benign subconscious allows us to find meaning in a positive and constructive way. Usually the sickness points to areas in our lives which need improvement or change. A technique that is useful "to connect" with the subconscious when we are not well and to find the meaning of our sickness is to focus on the symptom or pain while hypnotized. The symptom is seen then as alive, and a conversation starts with the symptom to find out *what it is trying to tell us*. If the answer does not appear immediately, we should relax more and try again. If it is still not forthcoming we should leave ourselves open to the answer from within us by requesting the part in us responsible for the symptom to let us know *what it means and how it is trying to help us*. Its answer, we ask, should come to us at any time: in our dreams or as a mental flash when we are doing ordinary things like driving the car, waiting in line, and so forth.

When the answer finally comes, a process of integration takes place. Parts in us which were neglected, denied, or abused are owned and cared for again. This facilitates healing because the symptom is no longer needed by our subconscious to force us to face aspects of ourselves we were ignoring. To repeat, this New Hypnosis technique presupposes that we do give our sickness medical attention if it is needed, while proceeding in the manner I am describing. I want to emphasize that the puzzle of the physical symptom is resolved more easily if we avoid asking *why* and stay with *what* and *how*, as indicated above. The why questions stimulate our conscious, logical mind at the time we need to communicate with our right-hemispheric, experiential, subconscious mind. By insisting on *what* is happening and *how* the symptom reflects something important to us, it is easier to connect with that part of us of which we are not aware.

The answer to our question about the symptom may create great conflicts in ourselves. The same truth that ultimately makes us free often creates acute pain in the process of inner liberation. However, the first step to inner freedom, to self-integration, is possible to take by means of our illness or sickness. This is a way of taking advantage of the Doctor within. Others call it the inner adviser (Bresler, 1977), spiritual guide (Jaffe, 1980), inner healer (Samuels and Bennett, 1974), or the healing mind (Oyle, 1976). The Doctor within can open the door to the mystery of our illness or sickness. By so doing, it releases the healing mechanisms of the body so we can return to normal healthy living and functioning.

One naturalistic way of taking advantage of the living Doctor within us is by following the OLD C model, paying special attention to the somatic elements. The somatic techniques described in Chapter 3, especially somatic bridge and subjective biofeedback, are direct means of activating the Doctor within. The following excerpt is taken from a session with a 38-year-old man who had been referred because of hypochondriacal obsession. At the point in the sixth session, he had improved "more than 50%" in his own evaluation. He had visualized his Doctor within as a woman.

Pt.: I can't help it. In spite of the great improvement, I still get worried when I don't feel well. I think whatever I have is very serious. (Patient was having a slight pain on the right side of the neck.)

DLA: You know how to handle this. Connect with your Doctor within. OK? Relax first, just like that . . . your eyes closed and letting each breath bring you closer to your very own living Doctor within. Let her come to your aid. She knows what the symptom is trying to tell you. Are you getting with it? (Patient nods head.) Focus now on your pain. Let the Doctor within you give your pain a personality, a life of its own. You still with me? (Patient nods head once more.) Now you can talk to your pain directly. OK? Ask it what it's doing there. Tell it you are noticing it and want to pay attention to it. Is there a message in its presence there? Take your time. Ask: Can I get rid of it? How? What should I do to get rid of it? Listen to your inner voice. Your doctor within is at work this very minute. Ask the same questions again. Can I get away from this pain now? How can I do it? What must I do to stop this pain?

Pt.: Somehow I feel I must trust my inner self more.

DLA: Say that to yourself. Repeat it again and again in different words. I must trust my inner self more.

Pt.: Yes. I want to trust my Doctor within. This pain is nonsense. I know I am not sick. It's just my worrying. It makes the symptoms.

DLA: Stay with this. Take your time.

Pt.: (silence, relaxed attitude, concentration). I want to trust my Doctor. She knows me. She knows what's good for me. She has been taking care of me for a long time. (big smile) Yes, I can trust her. My pain is gone (touching the area of the neck where he had the pain).

DLA: The pain is gone. It seemed to have come to remind you of the need to trust your inner Doctor. Thank her now for this communication.

Pt.: (silence, but relaxed concentration with a peaceful smile) Yes, I am grateful. (silence)

DLA: Now check with your whole being. Is everything at peace? Is every part of you pleased with this experience? Take your time to check it.

Pt.: (broader smile) Yes, I feel fine. My whole self is OK. I feel great!

DLA: Before ending now, say to yourself that you'll use this same technique in the future, anytime you start feeling pain. You'll take a few moments to contact your Doctor within and learn from her how to handle your pain.

Agreeing with Jaffe (1980), I believe every person has an inner adviser living within him or her. At some level we all know how to heal ourselves. Once we have uncovered the truth, we must find the courage to act on it. But the New Hypnosis, with these naturalistic techniques, is a great help to start this process of honesty with oneself.

CONCLUSION

Early in this chapter I pointed to the reluctance of the medical establishment to integrate the view of inner self-healing with the marvelous technology it has achieved in the last few years. Dismissing the mind makes healing artificial and unnatural. Harmony of all aspects of our humanity and integration should be the goal. The New Hypnosis provides powerful tools to achieve these goals. And the fact that these tools are naturalistic, as well as easy to learn and apply, provides therapists with the opportunity to integrate the body in their work. Medicine ignored the mind and soul of humans, but most psychotherapy has ignored the human body. The attention to the Doctor within—the use of the OLD C model which considers somatics among the essential aspects of communication between the patient and the therapist— will overcome the neglect of the body by therapists. However, this neglect of the body is by no means the invention of psychotherapists. In the Judeo-Christian tradition there is plenty of evidence of negativism about the body. Orthodoxy, whether Jewish, Catholic, Baptist, or Evangelical, has in common a sense of inhibition, fear, and prudishness about the body. In early Christian thinking it was a virtue to hate the body, to submit it to the spirit through penance, fasting, and physical pain. I hope we are in the midst of a change towards monistic holism: that the body will be considered the self as much as the mind is seen as the self. The techniques of the New Hypnosis will hopefully contribute to that holism.

Our inner healer refers to a powerful resource we all have as long as we are alive. It is the ability of the human mind to influence the physiological processes involved in healing and regeneration. The fact that our Western culture as a whole has neglected to "educate" this natural human power does not make it disappear. Some of the "miraculous" results obtained through the use of our inner healer may be more normal than we have been taught to believe—and consequently, to expect.

The current resurgence of interest in eniatric healing, both in religious and in scientific circles, points to the fact that a right-hemispheric attitude, in which belief prevails, is not that exceptional to normal behavior. In a religious atmosphere this belief is focused directly on a higher power. In scientific orientations the belief in this unique human resource of self-healing is enhanced and utilized for the benefit of the individual. The New Hypnosis, with its naturalistic methods, makes it easy to activate the inner healer in all of us.

Part IV

Applications

The two chapters in this last part present a detailed description of how I work using the New Hypnosis. It is unnecessary and tedious to transcribe verbatim every single exchange that took place in each session. I have tried to keep as much verbatim material as necessary to give the true flavor of the clients and their interaction with me; but I have also summarized certain segments of the sessions, while keeping my comments brief and nonspeculative.

These two vignettes are offered in the hope that the reader will be able to experience firsthand, as it were, the application of the New Hypnosis in clinical work, both in a system's case (which is my preferred way to work whenever this is possible) and in a clinical case with just one individual.

The two case illustrations chosen come from different times in my practice. It was revealing to notice clear consistencies in my work, in spite of the six years that had elapsed between the two cases reported here.

8

A "Model" Family

The following case concerns a family in desperate need of help when they contacted me. However, they were skeptical because they had been in therapy years earlier for some problems of discipline with their oldest son, but to no avail. As it turned out, the "family therapist" was a state licensed psychologist whose academic degree was in experimental psychology and who had not taken any subsequent formal training in either psychotherapy or family therapy. Not knowing about the therapist's professional background, the family attributed their disillusionment to the failure of family therapy.

GENERAL BACKGROUND

The Z family consisted of a 62-year-old father, a 58-year-old mother, a 25-year-old daughter, and a 27-year-old, married son who did not attend the family hypnotherapy sessions because for the last two years he had been living in another state. The mother made the initial telephone contact and said, in a very upset voice, that "something horrible has happened in our family," but refused to explain any more over the phone. I shall return to the presenting problem in the section on the first session. The daughter, Daisy, was a social worker in a municipal agency

143

dealing with derelicts and other desperate and often hopeless cases of human suffering. She lived in a big city in a modern condominium. Her parents lived in one of the wealthiest suburbs. The father was a successful administrator of a private international foundation which required frequent travel to the West coast of the United States, as well as to European cities. The mother was a wealthy matron, involved in many charitable and community enterprises. The parents were very religious, keeping the traditions of Judaism faithfully according to Jewish orthodoxy. As a matter of fact, they were referred to me by their Rabbi, to whom the mother first went to consult about this crisis. Because of his recommendation, they had agreed to try family therapy once more. Daisy (her original name had been Rachel but she had changed it to Daisy when she was a teenager) was outspoken against "the hypocrisy of organized religion, Jewish, Catholic, or Evangelical" and refused to participate in any of the religious holidays.

I asked the mother over the phone whether her husband and daughter were interested in family therapy themselves or whether they were coming only at her prompting. She responded, "Yes. They want to see you. The problem is mainly between them."

FIRST SESSION

The "something horrible (that had) happened in our family," as the mother had put it, occurred about a week earlier when the father had been at a nightclub where nude dancing girls entertain the clientele. One of the dancing girls was none other than Daisy. In embarrassment, he had left the premises. The following Sunday Daisy visited her parents and brought up the incident in front of both of them. The mother reacted with great anger, hurt, and confusion. She was incensed at both her husband ("What's he doing in a place like that, the old goat?") and her daughter ("A nice girl from a fine Jewish home, acting like a prostitute, in a sleazy place like that!"). The daughter, calm and amused, explained that she did not see anything wrong with her "moonlighting," that the nightclub in question was an elegant place with "respectable and classy customers," that this was for her a form of therapy in order to forget all the misery of her job, and that dancing in that setting gave her a great sense of power and control. She added, "If you were not such a tight-ass about everything, I would have told you about it a long time ago," and held her smile and her stare on the mother.

The father, on the other hand was humiliated, embarrassed, and angry ("That I had to look at my own daughter naked. She's disgusting"). The following is a verbatim transcript of the next part of the session. (The notation " . . . " indicates a pause.)

Mrs. Z: You talk about disgusting! What about you? What were *you* doing in a sleazy place like that?

Daisy: (interrupting and angry) I told you that it is not a sleazy place.

Mrs. Z: You hear her? She's proud of acting like a prostitute? All the money we spent on dancing lessons for her, for this? What do you say, Doctor?

Daisy: Yes, Mother. I'm not like you, thank God!

DLA: Let's get to the point and see what we can do about it. Mrs. Z, could you, please, get inside of you and connect with your anger?

Mrs. Z: What do you mean?

DLA: Just imagine yourself letting all your anger out at your daughter. *Pretend* . . . you are letting her have it, in your mind. Yell, hit her, throw things at her . . . And you, Dad, and you, Daisy, also get in touch with your own anger.

Mrs. Z: This is ridiculous. We came here to talk, not to play pretend games.

DLA: You are absolutely right, Mrs. Z, but to talk in a meaningful way, you all must be in touch with the anger you're feeling.

Mr. Z: You mean, we should imagine hurting each other?

DLA: No, not necessarily. You should let the anger come out in your imagination, so we can talk about it later. Let the anger come out *in your mind*.

Mrs. Z: What are we supposed to do?

DLA: Just close your eyes. You too, Daisy, please. Good. Now, acknowledge that you're angry . . . Check the anger in you . . .

Mrs. Z: (interrupting) I know why I am angry, because . . .

DLA: (interrupting) Yes. You know the reasons. Now let's recognize the *quality* of the anger, what form it takes. . . . Close your eyes, now . . . great . . . just like that. . . . Now, connect with your anger. . . . Imagine . . . you are expressing your anger at your daughter . . . at each other. . . . Look at it as if you were watching a very real movie of yourself . . . fighting . . . furious . . . no stops at all. . . . Everything comes out . . . like an explosion. . . . Keep breathing gently and . . . peacefully . . . but with each breath . . . get closer . . . to your anger. . . .

I kept talking in this manner for about 10 minutes, while the three of them kept their eyes closed and appeared to follow my instructions. I kept asking questions like, ''Are you with it?'' ''Are you getting into it?'' and ''Still OK?''

DLA: Now, slowly, let yourselves come back to the ordinary mental channel once more. . . . No rush, though. . . . But you are coming back . . . to the ordinary way of using your mind . . . so we can talk about it, as Mrs. Z said. . . .

Mr. Z: That was interesting, Doctor . . . I guess, I'm somewhat angry at my wife too . . . I didn't know this. I guess we must be honest here. I'm angry at you, Alice . . . I'm sorry, but I am. . . . You can be difficult, you know?

DLA: What came up during the mind exercise you just did, Mr. Z?

Mr. Z: Well, I don't know . . . I guess I have to think about it. . . .

DLA: Perhaps you do. We'll come back to it at another time. Is that all right with you?

Mr. Z: Yes, I guess so.

DLA: What about you two ladies?

Mrs. Z: Don't call her a lady!

Daisy: There we go again! Yes, I was furious at you. I saw myself screaming my head off. I was beating you up and screaming.

Mrs. Z: You see, Doctor. Always disrespectful. Since she was a little girl, always rebellious. Never wanted to do things with the family.

DLA: What was your pretending like, Mrs. Z? Remember this was all pretending.

Mrs. Z: Well, Doctor. I felt how angry I am at her. I guess I'm disappointed. She was always so different from Jeff (her son, Daisy's brother). You know, at times I thought they had made a mistake in the hospital and had given me the wrong baby.

Daisy: Go ahead, now, I'm not your daughter. So what do you care, if I'm not your daughter? (Her eyes are moist now.)

DLA: Let's stay with the mental pictures you had a minute ago. You want to finish, Mrs. Z?

Mrs. Z: Well, I saw myself crying and yelling. . . .

DLA: Were you saying anything?

Mrs. Z: I was yelling, "You are not my daughter. You are not my child."

Daisy: Yes, I know how you feel. I'm not what you want me to be.

DLA: And you, Daisy? Anything else?

Daisy: Just what I said. I was angry at her, beating her—no respect, as she says. I was angry—I guess I *am* angry—at the way she treats Dad. It's sad.

Mrs. Z: Stay out of it, you slut. It's none of your business how Dad and I treat each other.

DLA: I suppose you're right, Mrs. Z, but let Daisy finish.

Daisy: Forget it. You can't talk with this woman. . . .

DLA: You are all upset, but this is only natural. . . . Go back inside you and now do something different. Imagine now your anger again, but not directed at each other. Just pure, naked anger. Let it come out in your mind's eye. It may appear as a volcano, or as a fire, or as a storm, or as an explosion, or as something different. . . . Close your eyes again, please. Get into it, now. . . .

Mr. Z: Excuse me, Doctor. I don't think Alice and Daisy should be so angry at each other.

Mrs. Z: The eternal peacemaker! Yes, I'm angry at her.

Daisy: And I'm angry at her.

Mrs. Z: And I'm angry at you, Joe.

DLA: Let's get back to the naked anger. We'll talk later . . . all right? . . . Close your eyes and imagine . . . your own per-

sonal anger . . . wearing itself off. . . . Let a mental image . . .
for your anger . . . form in . . . your mind. . . . A clear image
. . . slowly . . . emerging . . . shaping up . . . in your mind.
. . . Stay with it for a while. . . . Let your anger . . . come . . .
all out . . . wear itself out. . . . Stay with it until nothing's left
. . . and you . . . are relaxed . . . exhausted perhaps . . . but
relaxed . . . quiet . . . tranquil . . . cleansed of your anger. . . .

Again, I continued this manner of talk for a while. When I observed less tension in the three of them, I invited them back to
left-hemispheric activity.

DLA: What was your image of anger, Mr. Z?
Mr. Z: Very interesting, Doctor . . . I was surprised . . . I had
    a big atomic explosion, like the one in Hiroshima. . . . But,
    then, there was peace, quiet. No radiation or pollution, but
    quiet . . . I didn't even hear your voice for a while. . . . And
    I know I was not sleeping. . . . Then I saw in that solitude the
    image of my wife coming at me. . . . But—interesting, Doctor
    —I saw her the way she was when we got married . . . an ap-
    parition . . . beautiful and peaceful. . . .
DLA: And you, Mrs. Z?
Mrs. Z: I feel better now. I guess, Rabbi M was right. Your ap-
    proach is different. I apologize for what I said before and the
    way I acted.
DLA: It's all right. Thank you . . . what else?
Mrs. Z: I was first on a big cruise ship. Then there was a big ex-
    plosion, a very big one at that. Then everybody drowned but
    I found myself in an underwater city, with beautiful gardens.
    When you said to stop, I felt amazed. I wanted to stay . . . in
    my underwater city.
DLA: Well, you can always go back there when you're at home.
    As a matter of fact, you may try to visit your underwater city
    every day, to find peace there. . . . What about you, Daisy?
Daisy: I had a hard time getting into it at first, but somehow when
    you mentioned "naked anger" for the third or fourth time,

I saw huge icebergs, like mountains in the North Pole, and they were crumbling with great force and noise. Everything became flat and behind those mountains of icebergs I saw a beautiful place with lots of green grass and flowers and little animals. . . .

DLA: Let's look at each other's mental images. Any questions? Any comments?

Mrs. Z: I feel good about this. I never thought my anger could go away so quickly. I'm still angry but it's different. I'm not revengeful, I guess . . . I feel good about Joe seeing me coming to him like a bride. And Daisy? Isn't it strange? Her mental picture was so much like mine. . . .

DLA: What about you, Mr. Z?

Mr. Z: I'm still under the spell of that whole experience. Very interesting. . . . Yes, I liked them all. I guess Daisy and Alice were reconciling each other with their similar pictures, eh? . . .

DLA: And you, Daisy?

Daisy: I also feel very good. I'm sorry this damn thing happened. I'm sorry if you (looking at her mother) think I'm a slut. I know I'm not. I'm not angry at you. I know we are different. Different life values. Different tastes. My dancing is a good thing for me. I love my body, I'm proud of it. (looking at me) Narcissistic, you would say, I suppose. And I don't see anything slutty about it. I don't tell the people at the agency because I'd lose my job but I *am* proud of it.

Mrs. Z: I guess we *are* different. . . . We can still love each other . . . I don't understand you, but I'll try. . . .

Daisy: Just accept me as different. Don't try to understand me. That's not as important as accepting me for what I am.

Mr. Z: The fact that both had similar mental images, I guess, means Daisy is not that different from Alice. At least her images . . .

DLA: . . . are similar to her mother's. Perhaps it's genetic. . . . Now, let's see if you can resolve this issue. There *was* a crisis. Dad here was surprised he was angry at Alice and will think about it. Mom here expressed her anger and disappointment.

Both Dad and Daisy had let her down. And Daisy asserted her right to live her life according to her best judgment. How do you think we can close this issue?

Daisy: I don't think it's my issue anymore. They should work this out, their anger at each other.

DLA: What do you think?

Mr. Z: You are the doctor.

Mrs. Z: (Nods assent.)

DLA: I believe Daisy is right, to a point. We should meet again without Daisy, at least once. Then before we finish therapy, we should see each other all together. Before we meet again, Mr. Z, think about your anger at your wife and try *not* to deny it. It's normal to feel angry at the people we love. . . . You, Mrs. Z, try to focus on what's good in your marriage, what you like about your husband. Do it in your underwater city, enjoying great inner peace. Make a list. . . . And Daisy, you'll have a vacation from therapy but I'll let you know when you should come back. Is it clear?

With the general assent, the session was ended and a new appointment was made for the following week. Before saying goodbye, I asked each to repeat to me his or her assignment, believing that the family should leave the therapy session with a clear understanding of what actions to take.

Comments on the First Session

The session started with open hostility. Had I let it go on in that vein, it probably would have taken more than one session to reach the point the family reached in this first family hypnotherapy meeting. After getting the general facts of the crisis, I had defined the two main issues: 1) the problems (not yet identified) between husband and wife; and 2) the reaction to/interpretation of the daughter's behavior on the part of the parents, especially the mother. There were other secondary issues, such as the possible jealousy/reaction formation of the mother towards the daughter. The decision to be made very early in the session was *where to focus*. It was clear in my mind that the anger was to be addressed first.

The entry point for therapeutic intervention came when, after the main facts were in the open, mother and daughter were ready to start a fruitless argument and the mother turned to me ("You hear her? She's proud of acting like a prostitute"). The useless exchange would have proceeded as it had begun, with irrelevant facts from the past brought up by the mother ("All the money we spent on dancing lessons," etc.). I ignored the exchange and stayed with the anger, inviting the mother to stay with it. Then I realized that it would be helpful for father and daughter to do the same and extended the invitation to both of them. The mention of *pretending* in order to describe the self-hypnosis work about to begin was an unfortunate choice, as the mother's comments about "playing pretend games" demonstrated. Since the mother had stated that they had come to talk, I agreed with her, clarifying *the quality* of verbal exchange by using "my method" in order to make the talk more effective.

At this point, the father's request for clarification was taken literally as such, without speculative interpretation of covert hostility towards his wife and daughter. Similarly, the mother's request for further instructions, even after my detailed explanation of what to do, was not taken as resistance, and a directive to close their eyes was firmly given. Later, ending the first segment of hypnotic work, I referred again to "Mrs. Z's intention to talk." Mother (resisting again?) mentioned "reasons why she is angry," and without arguing or disagreeing, I insisted on getting into this mind exercise. Slowly the three involved themselves in the mental activity. My directions at that point were given very slowly, with long pauses, and getting feedback from them.

After this first segment of hypnotic work, I invited the family to process the experience, addressing myself first to the father and thus honoring this family's strict hierarchical structure and avoiding unnecessary (unconscious) resistance if, by my actions, I had implied that this family had no "head of the family." My response to the father's comment ("You'll come back to it another time") was an imbedded message about his avowed ignorance of what he had experienced a moment ago.

The mother's reaction when I referred to her and the daughter as ladies, the daughter's response, and the mother's retort could have started a fight which, paradoxically, would have distracted them from the anger which I was helping them to deal with. Previously also, when the mother, quoting herself, said, "You are not my daughter," Daisy, by not taking it personally, helped to avoid another detour and to stay with the anger, rather than with current manifestations of it. This type of exchange was in danger of getting into petty details, confusing past incidents with the current issue. I ignored the mother's attempt to bring me to her side and went back to the "pretending exercise." This also confirmed for me the decision, already formulated in my mind, of seeing the couple alone in the next session.

The meaningful interchange among the three family members continued in the session. This made it possible for them to own their anger at each other and to get in touch with it. Rather than appease them, I invited them to get rid of the anger by suggesting the next hypnotic piece of work by using mental images in order to let the anger spend itself.

My reference to "naked anger" which Daisy used in her imagery, as she explained later, was a manifestation of my countertransference. Daisy was a very attractive young woman, with a perfect figure, a beautiful face, and a melodious voice. A part of me was distracted with the image of her naked dancing as a go-go girl and, even though I was ignoring it consciously, my subconscious found a way of bringing it up.

The father, "always the peacemaker," as the mother said, tried to do away with the hostility between mother and daughter. But I, because of my subconscious concern with their "naked anger," went back to the proposed mind exercise. Finally, they became involved in it and the results were beneficial, as their report of it indicated. In spite of the father's intellectualization, he entered quite thoroughly the imaginative work and acquired new information about himself by means of it. In the following sessions, his image of peace after the atomic explosion, as well as that of his wife in the underwater city, will be used to explore their relationship.

This hypnotic work benefited Mrs. Z also, to the point that she felt the need to apologize for her earlier expressions of anger and for her having questioned my "pretend games." After she described her image, I took the opportunity to instruct her in the therapeutic use of her peaceful image at home which I connected again, at the end of the session, with her behavioral prescription.

Daisy's report exonerated my "naked anger" image. When I asked for reactions to each other's images, the mother was effusive and tried to approach Daisy emotionally by remarking on the similarity between their two peaceful images during the hypnotic exercise just completed. The father felt good about this similarity also. At the end of this exchange, based on their mental pictures, I returned the responsibility of "resolving this issue" to them, to counteract the appeal to authority they had employed a couple of times before and, again, a few times later when they addressed themselves to me.

I ended the session with clear and concrete behavioral prescriptions for husband and wife. By not assigning any prescription for Daisy, I was validating her lifestyle without assuming unconscious dynamics of narcissism or exhibitionism, of penis envy or castrating drives, and without getting into any political issues of women's exploitation or the emphasis on the female body as merely a sex object for men. The reason to avoid these fascinating lateral issues, either subconscious or sociopolitical, is that neither Daisy nor the parents had come to me in order to explore them.

SECOND SESSION

The couple and I next met five days later due to one of Mr. Z's overseas trips. Mrs. Z, who in the first session had been dressed in accordance with her mood, plainly and in dark colors, without makeup or jewelry, was now dressed as if she were going to a party: a bright-colored dress, and much jewelry and makeup. She started the session.

Mrs. Z: What do you think of Daisy, Doctor? At times I think there is something wrong with her, with her mind, I mean. What do you think?

DLA: Did you two have a chance to discuss what we talked about last time?

Mrs. Z: Well, Daisy has always been a problem. So different from Jeff. She . . .

DLA: (interrupting) Tell me what went on between both of you after the first session. Mr. Z?

Mr. Z: That's the problem. My wife keeps talking of Daisy, comparing her with Jeff. But we have to talk about ourselves.

DLA: Each one of you had something to do since our last meeting. How did you do? Mrs. Z?

Mrs. Z: Well, I tried to go back to my underwater city, but I just didn't have the time. I've been busy . . . and so upset about this whole situation. Why is Joe going to those sleazy places, anyway?

Mr. Z: I did think about my anger with Alice, but I did *not* have a chance to talk to her. We hardly see each other. I'm home most evenings but she's always busy—meetings, committees, affairs. . . .

Mrs. Z: With all your travel, I have to keep myself busy. . . .

DLA: All right. In the next few minutes, you, Mrz. Z, can go back to your underwater city, and you, Mr. Z, can rehearse in your mind the conversation you'd like to have with your wife. Let's do it now. Just close your eyes, like you did last time, and follow my instructions, listen to my voice. Very well, just like that, breathing nicely, slowly . . . Mrs. Z, be back in your marvelous underwater city. Admire . . . the beauty of the place. Stroll gently through the gardens and . . . allow yourself . . . to feel good, really good. Mr. Z, you find yourself in a comfortable place talking to your wife. Where are you?

Mr. Z: In the den.

Mrs. Z: I can't get into it. It's not working.

DLA: It's all right, Mrs. Z. While Joe is in the den, you may relax
even more. Joe is imagining that he is talking to you and . . .
you can enjoy your breathing . . . feel the relaxation in your
shoulders . . . in your neck. . . . How is it going now?

Mrs. Z: Better now.

DLA: Enjoy your body . . . relaxing . . . all over. Check: Where
is it more relaxed?

Mrs. Z: My legs . . . my arms, too.

DLA: That's marvelous! You are doing so fine! Ask yourself, How
long will it take to be fully relaxed? . . . One minute? . . . Five
minutes? . . . While you, Mr. Z, rehearse the conversation you
want to have with your wife. Have it now. You are in the den,
in the midst of that talk right now. . . . Listen to your voice.
. . . And Alice is getting even more relaxed. Listen to her voice
in the conversation you're having now in your mind. . . . Be
aware of your good feelings. . . . In spite of everything, you
care for each other . . . there is a lot of good between the two
of you. . . . How are you doing now, Mrs. Z?

Mrs. Z: Better, fine (now showing all the indications of being in
a trance).

DLA: Are you still talking to your wife, Mr. Z?

Mr. Z: Yes . . . (also showing trance behavior).

DLA: Where are you, Mrs. Z, in your mind?

Mrs. Z: (smiling) My beautiful place . . . so gorgeous . . .

DLA: See yourself sitting someplace, an elegant bench, perhaps . . . and somehow there, you can listen to your husband.
. . . You'll connect with his mind in your mind . . . some mental form of communication.

Mrs. Z: I don't hear anything. . . .

DLA: Mr. Z, talk to your wife. Tell her some good thing . . . positive . . . now.

Mr. Z: Alice, we've been together a long time. . . . You are part
of my life. . . . Of course I care about you. . . .

Mrs. Z: (in an angry tone, still in trance) Yes, you care. . . . Those
sleazy places . . .

Mr. Z: Alice, I love you, but we haven't had sex in years. . . . I'm
not a man . . . with you. . . .

Mrs. Z: (submissive) I know . . . I just can't. . . . It's in the past.
. . . You don't touch me. . . .

Mr. Z: (opening his eyes and looking at me) I guess we *are* having a conversation after all.

DLA: Close your eyes again. Yes, you are talking. You are relaxed. Tell Alice what *you* would want.

Mr. Z: I'd like to be husband and wife again.

DLA: Say it again, with all your feeling.

Mr. Z: Yes, Alice. I want to love you again . . . fully. To make love to you . . . to be your husband in truth . . . in the bedroom. . . .

Mrs. Z: (with tears in her eyes) I . . . know. . . .

DLA: Mrs. Z, what do you say?

Mrs. Z: (in a rather childish voice) I want that too, but . . . I'm afraid. . . . I'm too old. . . .

DLA: Mr. Z?

Mr. Z: I feel sad. . . . She's not old. . . .

DLA: (interrupting) Talk to Alice, please, Joe.

Mr. Z: You are OK, Alice. Age is unimportant . . . I won't hurt you . . . I'm sorry about my affair, I'm sorry about the go-go club. . . . I still want you . . . but you must want me. . . .

Mrs. Z: (in her normal voice again) I'm still afraid, Joe . . . I guess we could try again . . . I guess I know you love me. . . . But you should show me.

Mr. Z: We must be alone . . . more.

Mrs. Z: I want to spend time with you . . . together . . . alone.

DLA: Perhaps you can look inside of you and see what concrete things you must do to start a good, full marriage once more. . . . Look inside you. . . .

Mrs. Z: . . . First thing . . . to sleep in the same bed, in the same room.

Mr. Z: I want that too. . . . We'll do it.

Mrs. Z: And we'll go out alone . . . no friends.

DLA: Imagine being out together, alone, the two of you . . . Where are you? What's happening?

Mr. Z: I guess . . .

DLA: (interrupting) No, wait. . . . Get into it, fully . . . first. Then, tell each other. . . .

Mrs. Z: A nice dinner . . . relaxed . . . alone.

Mr. Z: Yes, I like that . . . romantic . . . together. . . .

DLA: Go back to the bedroom. Sleeping in the same bed. How does that feel? Get into it first, feel it first . . . then tell each other. . . .

Mr. Z: It's good. . . . I like it.

Mrs. Z: I don't know. . . . It has been so long . . . I'm afraid. . . .

Mr. Z: I promise, Alice . . . I won't hurt you again . . . ever!

Mrs. Z: I can try . . . just try.

DLA: Let's go back to the dinner alone and being romantic.

Mrs. Z: That feels better. . . .

Mr. Z: No problem there. . . . It's good.

DLA: All right, then. Let's come back to the ordinary way of thinking. Slowly now. . . . When your eyes open, feel nice and relaxed.

(Both returned to left-hemispheric functioning at the same time and spent a little while reorienting themselves. Then we discussed what had happened.)

DLA: How are things now?

Mr. Z: I feel much better. We do have to make some changes. Drastic changes.

Mrs. Z: I'd like to start slowly. Perhaps go out together a couple of times. Then we can move in together. Joe can come back to the main bedroom. Then, we'll see what happens.

Mr. Z: (showing annoyance in his voice) How long will that take, love? (looking at me) She means sex, you know.

Mrs. Z: I don't know, Joe. You know I'm slow to change. We haven't been together, I mean, for over five years. What am I saying? It's at least seven years. First it was your snoring, then you had all your clothes in the other bedroom . . . always sleeping in different beds, even on trips, in hotels. How do you think I felt? Add to this the affair for two whole years. Now the dancing girls . . .

Mr. Z: (conciliatory) Let's not fight now. I understand. We'll start again. (to me) I guess it's never too late to start, eh, Doctor? (to wife) We'll start again. Tomorrow I cancel my meeting. Will you cancel yours? And I'll take you to the nicest restaurant in New York. It'll be a surprise.

Mrs. Z: That sounds better.

DLA: Both of you, check inside. How do you feel? Contact your feeling. Don't speak yet. Experience your feeling fully. Yes, close your eyes and . . . relax. It's as if you are courting again. . . . Get in touch with the feeling. . . .

Mrs. Z: (after about one minute) Yes, that's good . . . I feel good.

Mr. Z: You know, I had some difficulty getting into it, but then, all my annoyance was gone. It felt good . . . I felt loving towards Alice, towards you, dear. It was good.

DLA: I'll leave you alone now for just five minutes. And you tell each other that you love each other, that you want to start again. (Then I left the office. On my return, I continued.) How did it go?

Mrs. Z: I was sort of . . . embarrassed, I guess you could say. But I appreciate Joe's words. I guess I believe him. But I'm still afraid.

Mr. Z: (tenderly) I know, darling, I know. We'll both be patient with each other.

DLA: That sounds very good. Now, let's go over what you did—I mean, during this whole session. What are your plans?

Mrs. Z: Let Mr. Z speak . . . I'll cancel my meeting tomorrow.

Mr. Z: OK. I appreciate that. First, we'll start spending some time alone. Not as much socializing and affairs and events and such.

DLA: Concretely?

Mr. Z: Yes. I'm getting there. We'll go out for dinner alone. Once a week. When we can, more than once. We'll also have one evening for ourselves. Sacred! Then, when she's ready, I'll move back to the bedroom. It'll be strange, after all these years. Then, I hope, we'll be husband and wife again.

DLA: All right. It sounds great. What do you think, Mrs. Z?

Mrs. Z: Yes. I'll go along with that plan.

DLA: Do it that way, then. We'll make an appointment for two weeks. That'll give you time to start your plan. Hopefully by then you'll be ready for the next step. How does that sound?

Both: Sounds OK. Yes, that's a good idea.

DLA: Fine, so this is it.

With this the session ended and a new appointment was made for two weeks later. Both left in a mood of relaxation and good will. On the way out, I said, "Surprise each other. The best may still be waiting for you." Both smiled and said good-bye.

Comments on the Second Session

The goal for this meeting had been defined in the previous one: to help the couple talk about their marriage and what truly had provoked the anger they felt towards each other. Even though all the details of their emotional dissatisfaction were not discussed, the main elements emerged spontaneously. Without delving into those past circumstances, I tried to help the couple to establish behavioral goals and to become motivated to improve their relationship. My dogged insistence on communicating in the here and now paid off.

After reviewing the behavioral prescriptions given in the previous session and realizing they had not practiced them, I used the session to do now hypnotically what they had not done during the week. In spite of her initial difficulty, Mrs. Z finally was able to start relaxing and eventually to use self-hypnosis. At this point, it was possible for husband and wife to engage in an exchange which was long overdue. Doing this in hypnosis facilitated the interaction without the normal rational defenses of people who have not been open with each other for a long time. It is worth noticing that at one point Mr. Z reverted to ordinary consciousness, commenting that they were really talking. Not to lose the momentum of their experience, I led him back to self-hypnosis and he returned to it without difficulty. It could be speculated that if I had engaged him in "rational" talk about the merits of this long overdue conversation with his wife, he would have lost the deeper meaning of the experience.

Shortly thereafter Mrs. Z had the beginning of an age regression, as her voice revealed, but it only served to activate the exchange between them: regression in the service of the ego, which has become an elegant formulation of the hypnotic experience, thanks to Kris (1952). I did not encourage her age regression,

however, for the same reason I did not encourage Mr. Z to comment rationally on the conversation he was having with his wife.
The exchange taking place then and there had a special momentum which could have been lost by either "distraction." Their
interaction, because it was a new experience after so many years,
had to be protected.

The result of this meaningful exchange between husband and
wife was Mr. Z's reassurance to his wife based on his feelings
of love towards her, regardless of his past transgressions. While
they were still in hypnosis, I suggested that they plan on the
needed changes to improve the marriage. Notice that Mrs. Z first
suggested sleeping together again, but then connected with her
fear of being hurt. Consequently, both decided on a "program,"
starting with dinners away from home but without friends and
with one evening weekly at home together. This plan of action
was confirmed later when they discussed their hypnotic experience. It became their own prescription, first to have relaxed dinners and evenings together and then to resume cohabitation. In
the discussion, and following the general OLD C model presented in Chapter 4, I suggested that they check again internally how
they truly felt about this plan to rekindle the marriage. After this
final check, Mr. Z reported that he felt "very loving" towards
his wife, and so I left them alone for a few minutes to express
these good feelings in private. This becomes more spontaneous
and natural than the therapist suggesting that they hold hands
or kiss each other in the presence of the therapist. Their exchange
was seemingly successful, although Mrs. Z referred once more
to being afraid. This issue will be picked up again in the following session. The final summary of the session emphasized the
concrete elements of the plan to be started immediately.

The goal of the session was accomplished. The couple had
been able to communicate in a meaningful way and to make concrete plans to revitalize the marriage. A time lapse of two weeks
before the next session was given in order to allow them time
to put their plan into action.

Looking back, it might be interesting to guess where the session might have gone had I allowed Mrs. Z to talk about her

daughter, as she attempted to do twice at the very beginning of this meeting. Instead, I pursued the goal I had in mind (namely, to open up a new method of communication between the spouses without speculating on Mrs. Z's motivations), ranging from a need to warm up, to manipulative maneuvers to bring me to her side, to resistance, to the real issue at hand.

THIRD SESSION

Two weeks later the couple had their next session with me. Both showed great eagerness to tell me how much progress they had made. Not only had they had three dinners alone in a relaxed, romantic setting, but they had decided to share the same bed after seven years of sleeping apart. Mr. Z had moved back to his wife's bedroom three nights previously and his wife was very happy about it. Mr. Z felt like a teenager, he stated, but very happy and proud of himself. They had not engaged in any sexual activity yet but "there is affection," as Mrs. Z put it. This progress seemed to me a bit premature. Consequently, I went back to her fears of being close and open after all these years of distancing and hurt, which had come up several times in the previous session. I suggested that to cement the progress made so far they might like to engage in another mind exercise. They agreed and we proceeded. What follows is a verbatim transcript of the rest of this third session.

DLA: All right, then. You know what to do. Close your eyes and take a moment to get centered . . . breathing gently, slowly . . . relaxing all over. . . . Now, go back through the years and select a few of the highlights of your marriage, as if you were looking at a family album. Just a few of the good moments . . . the positive times together . . . the times of peace, and happiness, and trust, and love. Are you getting into it? (Both nod yes.) Relive those good moments. Pick one first. Be there again. Still with it? (Yes nod from each.) Live that moment now. Be there. Feel good. All the good feelings . . . growing inside of

you . . . taking over the whole of you. . . . Are you there?
(Both nod yes.) . . . Now, move to the present, but hold on
to those good moments. . . . What can you learn *for now* from
those good moments? . . . Can you bring for today some of
the things you had . . . in those good moments? . . . Enrich
the now with some of the things . . . those feelings still here
. . . from the good moments in your life together. The virtues,
the resources, the wisdom. . . . Put together some things from
the good moments in the past . . . in the present. . . . Are you
doing it now? (Yes from both.) Enrich the present, yes? (Yes.)
with the past. . . . Some feelings, attitudes, from the past are
still useful today. . . . Are you into it? (Yes.) . . . Put them
together with what you are today. . . . Use what you've learned
from your good past to make today better. . . . Use your
wisdom. . . .

This manner of talk went on for several more minutes. After
they had left the hypnotic state of mind (out of trance), we discussed their scenes from the past. Both husband and wife remembered several important landmarks in their marriage, showing
an agreement which surprised both of them. I asked them what
they could bring to the present from those incidents from the
past, and to help them make that selection I led them back into
self-hypnosis. For the next few minutes I suggested they let their
inner mind choose any attitude or behavior from the past that
might still be useful in the present and future.

DLA: While you are reviewing very quickly those good moments
from the past once more, let some attitudes emerge . . . which
can still be used today . . . to make things happier between
you. . . . Briefly reviewing good moments between you . . .
and out of those moments you extract something from your
feelings, your attitudes, your wisdom. . . . You can transfer
to a current situation. . . . Do it gently. . . . How a virtue from
the past can be used again now. . . .

These suggestions were continued for a while. Then, out of
hypnosis, we processed what some of these ''virtues'' from the

past were. Once more, they agreed on several important attitudes, such as verbally exchanging impressions of their day in a relaxed "happy-to-be-together" frame of mind, as Mrs. Z put it. Then I continued.

DLA: To be sure that this enrichment takes place, let's rehearse situations which might imperil the enrichment. (Both agreed nonverbally.) Go back, then, and try to pick up in the past situations that made you feel distant from each other. Focus on one at a time . . . difficult situations for the marriage. . . . Look at them in your mind's eye. . . . Are you getting there? (Both nod yes.) You felt bad about each other, distant, unloving. . . . Get into these situations. But don't get into them too much. Look at them from a distance now. . . . Study one of those situations in slow motion. . . . Discover . . . if the other does something . . . says something . . . or doesn't do or say what you expect. . . . Discover what it is that makes you feel distant from the other. . . . Is the other triggering something in you? . . . Is there a pattern of behavior and reaction . . . through the years? . . . Something the other does triggers bad feelings in you . . . or something the other doesn't do? . . . Look at the whole picture and discover . . . what it is. Are you with it? (Both indicate yes.)

Again, in this instance, I continued suggesting that they find some cues given by the other that started a negative reaction in them. After hypnosis we discussed this and several behaviors were identified. For instance, 1) Mr. Z acting as if his wife were dumb (as she expressed it) and, in his words, 2) her fussing over him without asking him whether he needed it or not. Even though they brought up other such behaviors, I invited them to stay with those two just mentioned and to be as concrete as they could manage. Self-hypnosis was used again in order to find more satisfying behaviors for the future.

DLA: Imagine a situation in the present when Joe treats you as if you were dumb. And you, Joe, imagine a situation when Alice fusses over you. . . . Can you zero in on one such in-

stance? (Both nod.) . . . But this time, you . . . both of you react differently to that situation. You don't let it get to you, but
do something effective about it. You handle the situation. See
yourself doing it. Experience yourself doing it. You use your
inner wisdom, built throughout the years . . . your inner resources from the past, to handle the situation without being
upset. You are in control. . . . Can you see it? (Both nod yes
repeatedly.) You seem to be very convinced you can now handle a bad situation. Do you? (Both indicate yes.) . . . Go over
it once more, to really be sure you can do it without any difficulty. Take a moment to do it. . . . All right? Then you are satisfied that it's going to be all right? . . . You may come back
to ordinary consciousness and we'll discuss what happened.

Husband and wife felt that this last practice had been useful
and requested to continue therapy in order to discover "more
of those things we do to each other to trigger the wrong reaction," as Mr. Z stated.

Mrs. Z: To rehearse, as you call it, the new way of reacting was
very helpful. You know what I saw myself doing? First time
in my life, mind you. Saying he's full of it! Sorry, Joe. I said,
"He's full of it. He's all wet. He's wrong," and so on. Finally, Joe is not the know-it-all. All of a sudden. But I love you,
Joe. I'm sorry.
Mr. Z: I know. I'm not offended. In fact, I'm glad—really—that
you see me for what I am. It's a relief! . . . I need your love
as a woman and companion, not as a mother or as a helpless
little girl.

With this, I asked them, as a behavioral prescription, to pay
attention, individually and together in their private moments,
to good memories from their long life together and to find out
what they could learn from the past to enrich the present, as they
had done in the session. In this way, new behaviors could emerge,
as Mrs. Z's assertiveness had emerged in the session with me,
to further enrich the marriage.
    Finally, we made arrangements for the next session together

with their daughter and, "if things are resolved," I added, "We'll
let Daisy graduate, at least for now, and we three will continue
working together, as we did today." They were pleased with this
plan. On the way out, Mrs. Z said to me, with a big smile, "The
good of the past to make the present better, eh?"

Comments on the Third Session

The behavioral prescriptions agreed upon during the previous
session had been practiced. In fact, the couple had progressed
faster than expected by moving back into the same bedroom after
years of sleeping apart. The first mind exercise they practiced during the session was directed at making sure that their changes
were not premature. I started by helping them to focus on positive experiences during their long relationship as husband and
wife. The rationale for this was to give them an experiential conviction of the positive feelings existing in the marriage. Then I
instructed them to review the past in a positive light once more,
but paying special attention to those attitudes, etc., from the past
which could be helpful and enriching in the present. Only then
did I suggest focusing on "danger areas" which might exist now
and reviewing them "pretending" that they were handled constructively with some of those virtues they had practiced in the
good moments from the past.

The next step was to discover what, years later, Ritterman
(1983) would refer to felicitously as family hypnosis or nonconsciously using hypnosis on each other. I was interested in their
becoming aware of the behaviors of each which might have an
"inductive" power over the other. In other words, at this stage
I led them to become aware of the power they might have over
each other, without realizing it, to imperil the relationship. Once
they identified two of these instances (Mr. Z treating his wife as
if she were less intelligent and able than him; her being overso-
licitous of him, even when he wanted to be left alone), they again
rehearsed in hypnosis how to handle these situations in a more
satisfying and enriching manner. Finally, these situations were
reviewed again in order to reinforce the new behaviors.

In summary, six steps were taken in the session:

1) Positive highlights of the marriage were reviewed.
2) Special attitudes from those highlights were identified in order to apply them to current situations.
3) Negative situations which might imperil their present progress were identified.
4) More concretely, *specific* behaviors inducing a negative response in the other were singled out.
5) A positive rehearsal of situations similar to #4, above, was practiced.
6) A repetition of #5 was used to reinforce and solidify the new behaviors.

Because the couple realized the value of the above sequence, they requested to continue conjoint therapy and I agreed. We saw each other for six more sessions, though the fourth also included Daisy, as will be described presently.

It was touching to hear Mrs. Z so happy because she had been able to stand up to her husband in her mind, although at this early stage ("First time in my life, mind you") she was apologetic to her husband. However, his positive reaction gave her permission to be assertive. As behavioral prescriptions, I suggested continued practice at home of what they had accomplished in this session.

The reason for bringing in the daughter for our next meeting was to close the issue of the nightclub and also to help the mother realize that now she could have a more satisfying reaction to her daughter who had been and continued to be so rebellious. Mrs. Z's parting words, referring to making the present better, were an added indication of their motivation to be in therapy.

FOURTH SESSION

A week later Mr. and Mrs. Z and their daughter were on time for their session. Daisy had visited her parents the previous Sunday and, all agreed, it had been a most enjoyable get-together.

Mrs. Z stated that she had realized how much she had to be proud of in Daisy, even though they disagreed on many things. According to Daisy, that had been the first time since she had become a social worker that her parents had shown genuine interest in her work, wanting to know details and circumstances. "I realized," Mrs. Z said, "that Daisy is a young woman fulfilling her responsibilities with great care. She is not a little girl anymore and she has to live her life the way she sees fit." Mr. Z agreed and added, "It's funny. I guess I knew it all along, but now I really know it. And I am proud of Daisy." Mrs. Z rejoined, "I guess we are getting used to thinking positive. What we did in our sessions is starting to work."

I asked Daisy whether she had any requests from her parents. With an earnest smile, she said, looking at her mother, "If you could continue to enjoy each other without meddling—I mean, in my life—things will be very good." I pressed for a concrete request she might have.

Daisy: Just trust me, accept me, even though I don't lead the life you would like. I'm not married. I've given you no grandchildren, I know. At times I feel bad about it, for your sake. Guilt, I guess. I'm not as liberated as I want to be. I dance at the club, I don't practice religion. I don't even believe God has all those laws for us to live by. But I am your daughter. I am a decent person and I am happy with my life. Can you grant me that? (Both agreed cheerfully.)

DLA: What if your father or mother, out of old habits, do meddle in your life, as you say?

Daisy: I get furious, I withdraw, I don't want anything to do with them.

DLA: Can we now examine alternative ways of handling that?

Daisy: What do you mean? You want me to ignore it?

DLA: No, not necessarily. Could you, at the very first sign of meddling, simply *remind them* of this session or of all the ways in which they are proud of you?

Daisy: I guess I could, but I doubt that it will work.

DLA: What do you think, Joe and Alice, could the three of you agree on this?

Mrs. Z: I don't understand. What do you want us to do?

DLA: Next time you meddle in Daisy's life, as she said, she can remind you nicely of what you are doing and not get mad. And you agree now to take that reminder and stop the meddling right away. Daisy agreed to just remind you, knowing you'll heed her warning, so she does not get furious or withdraw.

Mrs. Z: I guess that would be nice. Yes.

DLA: Is that all right with you too, Mr. Z?

Mr. Z: Yes, I think it's a very good idea.

DLA: And you, Daisy?

Daisy: Oh, yes. I'd love it if it works.

DLA: OK. Let's make it work. Give me a situation that would infuriate you.

Daisy: (without hesitation and to her mother) Your asking me about my dates—who the guy is, what is his background. I wish you wouldn't.

Mr. Z: I've told you, Alice. It's not a good idea.

Mrs. Z: There you go again, Joe. I don't need your guidance.

DLA: Let's use self-hypnosis to correct that. Let's all imagine very vividly that scene. Daisy, you are visiting your parents and your mother, here, asks you about your dates. Now, using your imagination, you can go over this but, this time, you don't get furious. You just remind your mother and she stops. Would you like to practice this now? (All assent.) All right. Start the way you know. That's right, close your eyes and relax for a moment. Center yourselves. Think of the scene and, with every breath you take, make the scene sharper. . . . You are all at the house. Daisy is visiting. Feel the comfort of being together. You may be all talking about Jeff's latest phone call or letter. Everything is pleasant. . . . Be there, feel it. . . . Then Mother, without thinking, goes back to her old habit again and asks Daisy about her dates. . . . Take it from here. You, Daisy, remind your mother of this session. Hear yourself talking to her. Feel calm and relaxed. . . . Your mother's question does not have the same effect it had before. You remind her

nicely and she responds nicely. . . . Listen to her voice. Look
at her face. Feel good at what's happening. Feel proud of yourself. . . . And you, Mother, feel the good feelings towards
your daughter. Yes, you want to respect her decisions. Yes,
you want to see her as a responsible adult. Yes, you are proud
of your daughter. You are proud of yourself for having such
a great daughter. . . . You, Father, witness the whole scene
with happiness and pride. Get in touch with your good feelings.

The three of them responded well to this mind exercise and
we repeated it once more. Then I asked the mother to spend another moment checking what feelings or sensations in her may
possibly trigger her question about Daisy's dates. She started to
explain what she thought was the reason but I interrupted.

DLA: Do it the easy way you know now. Go inside of yourself
and relive what happens inside of you. Thoughts that come
or feelings . . . sensations in your body, memories. . . . What
happens inside of you before you ask that question?

(The mother spent about one minute in self-hypnosis. At the end,
in a quiet and slow voice, she spoke with her eyes still closed.)

Mrs. Z: I guess I think of myself when I was her age. . . . I know
Daisy is not me, but I feel inside that she should be married
already. I am also afraid I won't see the grandchildren. Jeff is
so far away; we see them only two, three times a year if we
are lucky . . . and here is Daisy getting to be an old maid.
Daisy: (laughing) Mother, we are different! I'll never be an old
maid, even if I don't ever marry. But, don't worry. One of
these days, I'll surprise you. I'll even marry a nice Jewish boy.
DLA: Go back to those feelings you experienced, Mrs. Z, thinking of when you were Daisy's age and feeling sad—afraid, I
should say—because you may not see Daisy's children. Focus
on that . . . feel the fear. . . . But add very clearly your own
conviction: "Daisy is OK. She is happy. That's what matters."
Say that to yourself again . . . and again . . . until you are sat-

isfied that your message is stronger than your negative feelings. OK?

After a few minutes, Mrs. Z opened her eyes and had a big smile. She commented on that message, "Yes, that she is happy is the most important thing. Everything else is selfish on my part." Daisy and her father were pleased with what had just happened, the latter reassuring his wife that she was not selfish.

The next issue I reintroduced was the incident that brought the family to therapy in the first place.

DLA: Let's now close the issue of the nightclub and Daisy's dancing there once and for all. Any feelings left?

Mrs. Z: It's in the past. I don't want to go back to it.

Mr. Z: Alice and I have talked about it and it is in the past. By the way, we are doing very well: dinner out and alone at least once a week and much more time together—weekends and one evening a week. We did talk about it and the issue is closed.

Daisy: Yes, I also feel it's good you (her parents) know about my moonlighting. I don't expect you to approve. I told you why I do it, what I get out of it. (with a kind smile) I have nothing to apologize for. I guess Father won't visit the club any more.

Mr. Z: (somewhat embarrassed) It's a closed issue now.

Daisy: It's not even an issue anymore. I feel good that it came out in the open. Not the way it did, but that it did.

Mrs. Z: Yes, we are moving ahead now.

DLA: So, we might as well finish with this. Last Sunday you had a nice visit. Correct? Go over it for a minute, resolving that you'll have many other visits just like that one. OK? (All three nod their heads in agreement.) So, go inside yourselves again and relive that visit. Great. Be there . . . get in touch with the good feelings again. That sense of peace and comfort with each other. . . . Say to yourself, "I like to feel this way towards my parents or towards my daughter. . . . I'll recapture these good feelings every time we are together . . . all the good feelings of loving each other and being together. . . . " Stay with this for a little while. . . . Then come back to the ordinary way of thinking, feeling relaxed and refreshed, ready to enjoy the rest of the day to the full.

We talked about this mental review. The experience had been positive for all. I recommended that they practice it by themselves at least once more and asked them to decide concretely when they would do it, not as a family but each on their own. Daisy expressed her positive feelings about the two sessions of family hypnotherapy and we said good-bye. The parents made a new appointment for themselves for the following week.

Comments on the Fourth Session

In this meeting the original problem came to a final resolution, although the couple continued in family hypnotherapy for five more sessions. This fourth meeting was definitely made easier by the pleasant experience the family had had the preceding Sunday when Daisy visited her parents. Their positive frame of mind with which they started the session revealed that the previous family hypnotherapy meetings had been successful and were producing good results. Both parents verbalized their recognition of their daughter as a young woman who had the right to make her own decisions about her lifestyle. This, to me, was one of the main issues underlying the presenting problem, the "leaving home" problem. To validate their statements, I could have used the technique of repeating the same phrase while checking their body reactions (see section in Chapter 3 on subjective biofeedback) but I chose to focus on Daisy (my countertransference still at work). Her "request" helped to confront the truth about the family's differences. This led me to suggest that they rehearse a family situation where the parents would again "meddle" in her life. When Daisy identified the issue of her dating and her not being married, I led them to practice mentally the new way of acting. This prepared the way for focusing on the mother's inner cognitions leading to her questioning Daisy about her private life. The mother realized her fear of not seeing Daisy's children and the way she identified with her daughter, as the dialogue shows. However, her awareness opened the door to asserting once more Daisy's decisions ("What matters is that she is happy").

Reviewing this part of the session, I realized that I could have asked them to repeat this mind exercise in order to firm the good feelings between parents and daughter even more. I did come back to it at the end of the session. When the mother, at this point, accepted Daisy as an autonomous adult I ignored her remarks about her selfishness in wanting to see Daisy married and with children in order to stay with the process that was going on. The experiential acceptance of the daughter as an adult was of paramount importance at the time.

The moment was then ripe for introducing for the last time the original presenting problem. Their reaction to this theme could have been seen as resistance, but I used it to foster progress. By accepting their probable self-deception about the issue being resolved and closed, I was able to move ahead without being forced to detour. As it happened, the issue of Mr. Z having visited that type of nightclub came up again in the sixth session when they dealt with the commitment to the marriage. In that session, Mr. Z felt free to talk about his sexual desires and the stimuli that aroused him. And at the seventh session the couple reported having started sexual activities once more after seven years of abstinence. They were both delighted with their ''new honeymoon.'' In retrospect, therefore, my not insisting on this issue during the fourth session turned out to be the right decision.

The last part of the fourth session, as I mentioned earlier, turned back to the good feelings the family had had during their visit the previous Sunday. I suggested that they take that visit as a model for the way they could feel towards each other, and Daisy finished with her participation in family hypnotherapy.

CONCLUSION

Going over this case, it is not difficult to discover the real issues underlying the presenting problem. These were, on the one hand, Daisy's leaving home and, on the other, the relationship of the couple. The first issue was handled in the fourth session, but the second one continued to be treated in subsequent sessions with the end result of a deeper commitment to the marriage and a noticeable improvement in their communication.

The incident that forced the couple to confront their distance and lack of meaningful interaction was the daughter's nude dancing and the father's embarrassing discovery of her "moonlighting." But this was circumstantial to the marital dysfunction. My hypnotherapeutic approach emphasized experiencing, not talking. Through it the couple moved at their own speed and made significant changes which truly improved their relationship. By following the basic OLD C sequence, I stayed always close to their own subconscious images, thus helping them become aware of their feelings. I simply assumed the role of guide and facilitator. This aided them in discovering new options and the solutions that emerged from their subconscious minds.

To me, the final criterion for successful therapy is that clients attain what they wanted to attain when they requested my services. In this case, it was obvious from the second session, at least, that their marital relationship was improving and was becoming more satisfying to both spouses. The daughter assumed the realistic place in the family system that she, at her age, had been denied by her parents' expectations.

I heard from this couple a year later, when Mr. Z called to request a financial statement for tax purposes. I had a chance to talk to both him and Mrs. Z on the telephone and they told me that things had continued to be satisfying and enriching for all of them. They added that both, individually, practiced self-hypnosis at least once a week for different purposes, such as nervousness or tiredness. This was a remarkable instance of generalization. The skills they learned during the family hypnotherapy sessions were applied to other areas of their lives.

They also reported that their weekly dinners by themselves and the evening together had become habits, and that they enjoyed doing this very much. Since we finished our hypnotherapy, they referred two other couples to me.

9

A Father Like
No Other

Having presented a case involving a social system in the previous chapter, I am now going to describe an individual case for whom a systemic approach would have been a distraction and a inelegant treatment procedure. This case took three individual hypnotherapy sessions.

GENERAL BACKGROUND

Jack called to make an appointment to see me for "hypnotherapy," referred by a neighbor of his, a psychologist who knows me. Because of a previous cancellation, I was able to see him the next day. Knowing that I am rather busy and on a tight schedule, Jack interpreted this as a good omen. The fact that I had answered the phone when he called added to his optimism.

He arrived five minutes early for his appointment and, when I invited him in 10 minutes later, greeted me with the comment, "Boy! Am I glad to see you, and that you were able to schedule me on such short notice." He was dressed neatly but casually in sedate colors. He explained that, after work, he had gone home to eat and change to more comfortable clothes than those he wears as a manager of a large plumbing supply store. At 28, his general manner was friendly and polite, and he was well-spoken and to the point. The following is the transcript of the first few minutes after the initial greetings and taking of essential data, such as address and phone numbers.

FIRST SESSION

DLA: What brings you here, then?

Jack: My father died a little over four months ago. We never got along. I hated his guts, like everybody else did. I still do. He was a nasty, ruthless, vicious businessman. People didn't count; only their dollar value. . . . Life for him was all business—the worst "dog-eat-dog" type. . . . I should be happy that he's finally gone, but I'm down—I hate the word depressed—lately. I wonder whether it's because of him . . . connected with him?

DLA: You want to explore your feelings towards your father, right? So, we must focus on your feelings—glad and down—and also on your father, your memories of him.

Jack: (as if thinking out loud) I guess that's it. . . . Yes.

DLA: Let's get to work, then. Are you sitting comfortably? Yes, you can recline the easy chair. Like that. . . . All right. If you would close your eyes and listen to me, we can start. Very well. Take a minute to relax and go inside of yourself, as it were. . . . Anything on your mind?

Jack: Just trying to relax.

DLA: Keep your eyes closed when you talk. It's less distracting after a while. In your inner mind, let yourself go to a very relaxed place, outdoors, beautiful, safe. . . . Sun shining, best time of year . . . superb weather. . . . What place comes to mind?

Jack: . . . Several. . . .

DLA: It's OK. Let them all go through your mind until you stay in one relaxed place. . . . Where are you now?

Jack: Meadow . . . beautiful . . . big mountains . . . very green . . . beautiful. . . .

DLA: Enjoy the place, the air, the quiet, the majesty. . . . Enjoy, be there completely. . . . You can see yourself there?

Jack: (Nods slowly.)

DLA: See yourself sitting in the position you are now. . . . Relaxing even more . . . And right there, in the beautiful meadow . . . surrounded by green mountains . . . you let yourself feel this down feeling you have experienced lately. . . . What happens?

Jack: (opening his eyes and with an anxious look) I was getting into it. I don't want depression.

I was helping Jack to do hypnotic work, or rather to get ready for it, and he was responding admirably well. However, when I introduced his current "down feeling" he opened his eyes and sat up as if startled. This was my mistake. My timing was premature. A way of avoiding this error would have been to use an old self-rating device with the help of the client's imagination. I could have asked him to picture a 12" ruler while he was enjoying his beautiful place, before getting into his depression. The numbers can measure either his relaxation or his readiness to communicate with his inner mind or subconscious. Depression is an "n-word" (words that contain negative messages). Even though I avoided using it, in his state of relaxation the mention of his "down feeling" connected with depression and he opened his eyes, stopping the relaxation. Perhaps Jack experienced a form of affective dissonance: starting to become relaxed on the one hand, and jolted by the memory of his current depression, on the other. Recognizing my error, I proceeded.

DLA: Go back to your meadow, please. Check whether you can be there again. . . . Pay attention to other details . . . nature sounds . . . birds . . . breeze . . . water running. . . . Enjoy. . . . Notice some wild flowers . . . their colors . . . the variety. Perhaps you see in the distance some rabbits or chipmunks. . . . You feel the gentle breeze on your face . . . the sunshine. . . . You smell the earth, the trees. . . . You taste the beauty of the place. . . . Are you into it? (Client nods yes.) Are you sitting there? (Yes.) . . . Enjoy being there, feeling very secure and happy . . . feeling very good and healthy. . . . While you are there, you may want to think of your life. . . . You want to think of your life? Yes? (Client nods yes.) You are alive, you feel alive . . . in contact with the beauty and life of this meadow. . . . Still OK? . . . Now, let your mind get in touch . . . with your feelings. . . . No effort. Just become aware of what's happening inside of you . . . as you are aware of everything that's happening in the meadow. . . . What's happening inside of you? Touch your soul . . . become aware of the life . . . inside of you . . . your feelings. . . . What's happening?

Jack: Shall I tell you?

DLA: Not necessarily. First, become fully aware of your feelings.

Jack: . . . I see my father. The father I always wanted . . . gentle, loving, encouraging. . . . But he changes into my real father . . . I'm afraid, angry . . . always. . . . We fight, yell, hurt . . . as always. There is no hope. . . . Oh, how I hate him. (now crying) I hate him . . . I can hear him, "You're just like me! What are you complaining about? You're just like me! You're *my* son. You have *my* blood! You're as much a son-of-a-bitch as I. Face it, kid. You *are* like me!" He keeps on yelling. It drives me crazy.

DLA: You are not like him *now*. He is dead; you are alive.

Jack: (ignoring my remark) I don't know what to do . . . I'd like to kill him. . . .

DLA: Let him yell himself out. You can . . . take it. And you can . . . change it.

Jack: . . . He's quiet now . . . but full of hate . . . I'm shaking. . . . Am I like him? . . . Maybe he's right. I'm like him. . . . Not in every way. . . . Yes, I have his same character but I don't like it . . . I don't want to be like him . . . I'd rather be dead.

DLA: Jack, face now the traits in your personality that *are* like your father. Let those traits come to your mind. . . . Like your father, you are . . . say to yourself, "Like my father, I am. . . . "

Finish the sentence in your own mind. . . . Do it again. . . .
You *are* like your father in many ways. Get into it: "Like my
father, I am. . . . ''

Jack: (intense silence of about two minutes) Yes, I know. I have
many of his qualities, but also I *am* different.

DLA: Yes, you are. Now, in your mind, let all those qualities,
the different ones, march past you . . . slowly . . . in slow
motion. . . . The things in you that are different from your
father. . . .

Jack: (quiet again; in intense concentration but starting to smile)
Not like him . . . at all.

DLA: Stay with them for a while. . . . (about one minute of
silence) Now, make a comparison . . . in your mind, as if you
were putting on the good qualities, like a piece of clothing.
. . . See two images of yourself and start dressing one image
of yourself with all the qualities in you that are *not* like your
father. . . . The other image of yourself *is* like your father. . . .
One like him; the other, not like him. Are you doing it? . . . Go
on until you're finished. . . . Now decide which *you* you want
to be. . . . Let the other image of you vanish, disappear. . . .
Stay with the image of the you you want to be. . . . The you
you want to be . . . the you you *can* be. . . . Stay with the you
you will be. . . . The you you know you can be. . . . Are you
with it?

This process took about five minutes, Jack visibly relaxing and
breathing very slowly. I asked him to stay with the good feelings and enjoy the self he was now choosing to enhance and let
flourish. Then I suggested that he continue this same mind exercise at home, practicing every day. After that we finished the
first session and made arrangements to meet again in seven days.
But, before we parted, I invited him to go over the whole experience he'd just had using self-hypnosis again.

DLA: As a final check, close your eyes again and review gently
the whole session you just had. . . . Check your body and let
it tell you how the session feels. . . . Any tension anywhere?

(slow head movement, indicating a no response) So, enjoy the good feeling and hold on to what you have learned today about yourself. . . . See yourself again as the you you want to be, you can be, you will be. Still relaxed? (Jack nods yes.) Finally, promise yourself to repeat this practice again, every day, until we meet next week.

Comments on the First Session

The first issue to highlight is that the goal of therapy was clearly defined from the very beginning. In Jack's case it was easy to do so. However, when the goal is not concretely stated, the initial task is to specify it. It should be noted that the therapeutic work starts right away. In other forms of therapy, Jack probably would have been encouraged to talk more about his father, to explain his feelings. My interest was in getting into right-hemispheric functioning as soon as possible, rather than to gather much initial information. The information about the client's life *that is relevant for change* will emerge spontaneously through inner experiencing rather than through direct probing, as the next sessions will demonstrate.

To make the transition from "ordinary mental activity" to self-hypnosis (as I explain frequently to new clients) it is necessary, especially in the beginning, to go through the initial phase of relaxation, centering oneself, getting into self-hypnosis or *induction* (if this latter term is used without meaning rituals or stereotyped techniques). In later sessions, this introductory phase is shorter or almost nonexistent, as we shall see in the second session with Jack.

When the goal is defined and when the client is ready (when he has "switched" from left- to right-hemispheric functioning), the item of concern always emerges, either directly, as in this session (his father "appears" when he is at peace, enjoying his imagery) or symbolically and in disguised form, as would happen in the second session with sexual material. When Jack got in touch with his father yelling at him, humiliating him and telling him that he was like his father, I mentioned two things: 1) the basic difference (''You are alive; he is dead'') based on his previous mental experience in the meadow where he had seen himself in contact with living nature; 2) my appeal to his inner strength and health (''You can take it; you can change it''). Even though Jack did not ostensibly respond to my first remark, he acted accordingly: He moved from the past to the future; he accepted change, the essence of life. Regarding my second comment, the following words from Jack were his response: ''I don't want to be like him.'' Later in the session I will build on this choice of Jack.

Before facing the traits in his personality that were like his father's, the client made a choice, reflected in one of those ''important statements'' mentioned in Chapter 4, ''I don't want to be like him.'' Notice how he ended up in that frame of mind, reassured by his own experiential work in hypnotherapy. By being encouraged to ''put on'' the positive traits in his personality, while recognizing the negative ones, Jack was able to repeat experientially his choice, ending by supporting his not-like-father self.

SECOND SESSION

Jack was on time for his 8:00 P.M. appointment, and started by saying he had done ''very well'' till the day before the session, but that the last two days had been ''terrible.'' Asked what doing well and doing terrible meant, he said:

Jack: I practiced every day and it was really getting to me. I don't have to be like my father. I already had rejected him when I refused to work in his great chain of stores and went on my own. Now I can reject him even more. But, better still, I can choose not to be like him.

DLA: Before you go on, Jack, check this rejection bit with your inner self, right now. Close your eyes, relax, and get into it: ''I don't want to be like my father.''

Jack: (relaxes, breathes slower) . . . It feels good . . . I *am* different. . . . His personality traits don't overtake me. . . . I can neutralize them. I won't become like him . . . ever! I feel it.

After this exchange, I asked him to continue with what he was telling me before about "feeling terrible." He answered that all the old fears had come back, that he had had nightmares about his father and himself fighting and shouting, as had happened innumerable times from his adolescence to his father's death. This had triggered the old depression again. At my invitation, he checked now how he was feeling, paying attention to his bodily sensations, not talking yet but getting in touch with his feelings. I reminded him, while he was doing this, of the way he had felt a few minutes earlier. This helped him recapitulate the positive feelings and he stayed with them again, savoring his decision not to be like his father.

DLA: Now that you feel so good, go to the way you felt yesterday and today. . . . Try to remember, to reexperience your feeling terrible. . . . Check what happens in your body. . . .

Jack: (smiling and relaxed) I can't feel terrible now . . . I feel good. . . . But I do remember how I felt yesterday.

DLA: Remember it then, relive it, and see if you learn something about yourself from reviewing the way you felt.

Jack: (concentrating, but still smiling) It was stupid . . . I let the old fears take over again. . . . No point in it . . . I *can* do it, I can be what I know I am. . . .

DLA: Again, then, let the you who is like your father go. . . . Let go of it.

Jack: The good me is stronger . . . I can let the other part of me go.

DLA: Do it now. Let the you you don't want shrink away, disappear. . . . Let it become so weak that it disappears . . . completely.

Jack:(after about one minute of silence) Yes, it's funny. I see my negative self shrink, vanish. . . . It feels fine. Next to it, I see the positive me . . . strong, alive, still growing. . . .

DLA: Enjoy this energy, growing, becoming stronger . . . taking over your whole being.

Jack: (frowning) It's getting too big. . . . Not so big, please. . . .

DLA: You can bring it back to the size you like . . . you feel comfortable with. . . .

Jack: Yes, it's not so big now. It feels OK. I can be that. . . .

DLA: Stay with it for a while. Become so used to the self you want
to be that the other does not have a chance any more. (Jack
stayed with it for a while, looking relaxed.) What are you
doing? . . . The self you want to be?

Jack: I'm with my lady . . . I'm enjoying her, not using her. . . .

DLA: Finish the scene. Be with her, the way you can be proud
of yourself.

Jack: Yes, happy . . . loving, sharing, sexual. . . .

DLA: Stay with it. . . . Once you're satisfied with this scene, let
your inner mind bring up another scene . . . different. . . .
What comes to mind?

Jack: At the store, with my men . . . helping them.

DLA: Again, Jack, you are there. See yourself acting fully like
you . . . unlike your father . . . nothing of your father left in
you.

Jack: Yes, it feels good. . . . Again, with my lady . . . really
mellow. . . .

Jack went back and forth between these two scenes several
times, reaffirming the person he wanted to be, strengthening the
image he wanted to hold on to. Practicing this in his mind, he
was weakening effectively the "father qualities" he wanted to
get rid of by strengthening those qualities he perceived as being
different from those of his father. The session continued in this
vein for about 15 minutes. At the end, we discussed his experience. He realized now that he had nothing to fear anymore
and felt that he had effectively let go of those qualities of his father
that he disliked in himself. Then we did a final check, hypnotically, to be sure that every part in his being was in agreement with
the previous experience during the session. This check, following the OLD C model, consisted of relaxing once more, using the
body as subjective biofeedback. While visualizing the self he
wanted, Jack was checking how his body reacted. As long as he

was relaxed and comfortable, he was encouraged to assume that his decision was right. If some tension had built up, the tension would have been focused on, in which case other issues may have appeared. He felt relaxed and satisfied and, with this, the session ended.

Comments on the Second Session

A few important details emerge right away in this session. Jack seemed to have started with a readiness to concentrate on the "failure" of the last two days, even though he had reinforced the gains made in the first session by practicing self-hypnosis at home. I channeled him to focus on those gains once more, rather than to concentrate on his failure. Only after he had recaptured the feelings which accompanied his decision not to be like his father did we move on to the "terrible" way he had felt the last two days. In doing so, he himself dismissed the fears of being like his father as ridiculous. To strengthen this perception of the like-father/not-like-father dichotomy, I introduced the two images of the self, one becoming stronger and the other weaker. I used the figure of speech of shrinking (an image he had not used before) and he responded to it positively.

According to the first step of *observation* in the OLD C model, the hypnotherapist should use the images offered by the client. However, when I introduced the image of *shrinking*, I was merely enlarging on his previous statement ("The good me is stronger. I can let the other part of me go"). From a visual perspective, if the "other part" is going away, it shrinks or becomes smaller and smaller until it disappears. In that same interaction I said, "Let it become so weak that it disappears," which was my nonconscious response to his previous reference to "the good self" as strong. Jack picked up right away on my new image of shrinking, which is a frequent occurrence with clients in this type of situation. Once clients are involved in right-hemispheric activity, they will accept new mental images suggested by the hypnotherapist, *as long as they are mere expansions of the ones they have used immediately before.* The receptive attitude of hypnosis, as Wick (1983) calls it, allows for this interplay between the client's and the hypnotherapist's subconscious minds (see Chapter 5 on the interaction between client and hypnotherapist).

Again, I introduced new concepts ("energy, growing, taking over your whole being"), all in harmony with what Jack was experiencing at the time. Then came that moment of mild anxiety when Jack said that the self he wanted to be "is getting too big." Leaving aside speculations about any possible sexual connotation, fears of homosexual attack, or concerns about penis size, I stayed with the images we were working with. This led him to see himself with his lady (a possible connection with the disguised sexual meaning of the previous exchange about "getting too big"). It could be speculated that the subconscious connection was made so smoothly because I did not force him to detour into sexual material when the first inkling of it appeared earlier. This paradox of ignoring the sexual connotation in order to allow its meaning to emerge spontaneously is in line with the postulate of noninterpretation inherent in the application of the New Hypnosis. Without being explicit, Jack refers to sex in his four adjectives ("happy, loving, sharing, sexual") and I encouraged him to complete the sexual scene with his lady.

The next image that ascended from Jack's subconscious mind was that of work, which was more like a new way of seeing himself acting differently than his father. Freud's *arbeiten und lieben* came to mind, as I watched Jack move between the two scenes that had emerged. He was going to be different than his father, both in work and in love. The original goal of therapy was being accomplished.

THIRD SESSION

Eight days later Jack came in, feeling very happy and encouraged. He said he knew now that he did not have to be like his father and reported that his depression had not appeared again. He talked about the callous ruthlessness with which his father operated, abusing women without any discretion or any regard for his mother. He also talked about his father "robbing people blind" when he could get away with it (and he could, because of his shady connections and corrupt friends in government), even being suspect of three murders, though charges had been dropped every time.

Since everything Jack had come to hypnotherapy for seemed to be consolidating in a healthy way, I suggested that he go back to his state of "feeling down" which he experienced in the first session. I told him that it could be useful to clarify this issue in order to immunize himself from such feelings in the future. He agreed to work on this, as the following verbatim excerpts show.

DLA: So, go back now to your self-hypnosis. Closing your eyes, just like that, and taking a moment to relax . . . to center yourself. You want to get in touch with that down feeling. . . . Check your body. . . . What happens there when you think of feeling down in connection with your father?

Jack: . . . All of a sudden, I'm very agitated.

DLA: Stay with that sensation in your body. Where is the agitation? . . . "Very agitated" . . . what happens in your body that you describe it as very agitated?

Jack: . . . All over, like a trembling. . . .

DLA: Don't avoid it. Go with it. . . . Let it build or let it weaken. Go with it.

Jack: (showing tension and frowning) . . . Sad . . . very sad. . . .

DLA: Allow any mental images to come up, any memories, any scenes. . . .

Jack: Dark . . . everything is dark . . . I'm lost. (The last statement was said in a childish voice.)

DLA: Stay with the darkness. Where are you?

Jack: Outdoors . . . night . . . cold, I'm cold . . . all dark . . . the wind. . . .

DLA: How old are you?

Jack: Ten, almost 11 . . . (still in a very childish voice) I'm not a big kid. . . .

DLA: What is your name?

Jack: Johnnie . . . I'm lost (now crying and agitated). . . .

DLA: Where were you before, Johnnie?

Jack: . . . With my mother.

DLA: Where?

Jack: . . . In the house . . . summer house. . . .

DLA: What happened?

Jack: . . . Daddy hit Mommy. . . . They were fighting . . . yelling. He hit her . . . he hit her hard . . . I run away . . . I'm
lost (still crying).

DLA: What happened next, Johnnie?

Jack: I hear Daddy calling me . . . I don't answer. . . .

DLA: And then, what happens?

Jack: He comes out with a big flashlight. . . . He doesn't see me.
I run . . . quietly. It's very dark . . . I'm cold. . . .

DLA: Go on, Johnnie.

Jack: . . . Then, I run. He hit Mommy. . . . She was crying. . . . I
hate Daddy, he's so bad. . . .

DLA: Are you still running, Johnnie?

Jack: No, I'm hiding . . . by the shack . . . I'm afraid. . . .

DLA: What happens then, Johnnie?

Jack: I hear Mommy. She calls me . . . I'm so happy she's OK.
Daddy is bad. . . .

DLA: What's your Mommy saying?

Jack: I hear Daddy. He says, "Leave him alone, the spoiled brat.
He'll come back. He's not stupid, the damn kid." He slams
the door, hard. . . .

DLA: And? . . .

Jack: But Mommy says, "You leave *me* alone." . . . I'm so glad
she's OK.

DLA: What else, Johnnie?

Jack: It's Mommy's voice, "Don't be afraid, Johnnie." I *hear* her.
"Everything is OK. Daddy won't hurt you. . . . "

DLA: So, what do you do?

Jack: "I'm here, Mommy." She hugs me. "Daddy won't hurt
you. He won't hurt *me* anymore either. It's OK now. . . . "

DLA: So, you're happy now?

Jack: (coming out of self-hypnosis, and speaking in his adult
voice) Boy, hah, that was quite a scene! You know, when we

went home, he was gone. He returned to the city that night. After that they separated. But, then, about six months later they were together again. That didn't last too long, maybe three years or so. That was the time when he would come around with his stupid girlfriends to upset my mother. Then, they divorced. I was about 15 at the time. She died when I was almost 20. I still blame him for her death. The divorce was sheer hell. He gave her incredible grief. Tortured her. She was not yet 45 when she died . . . I guess I'm still depressed about it . . . though, no. I've mourned my mother. It's only good feelings about her. . . . But him . . .

DLA: We were getting into your depression when you felt agitated and that, in turn, led you to that scene you relived just now. Go back inside of yourself and ask yourself how this scene is or was connected with your down feelings.

Jack: (smiling) You can use the word depression. I said that I hated the word because my father used to accuse me of being depressed—which, for him was very bad, since he had so much energy all the time. If he had only used it in a better way. He made a lot of money but no one loved him. But that's finished now. . . . What were you saying? Ah, the depression and that powerful scene I relived, yes. All right (closing his eyes and breathing deeply). . . .

DLA: Just gently, let yourself review how feeling depressed is related to the scene you just relived. . . . Don't figure out or analyze. Just let the thought come to you . . . the images, feelings, sensations come to you.

Jack: (relaxing more) . . . I guess I know. I never had a Daddy (and almost embarrassed) I'm sorry, I mean, a father. . . .

DLA: Yes, go on.

Jack: (now again in hypnosis) As long as he was alive, I hoped. . . . Someday, maybe . . . I could love him. . . .

DLA: But now he's dead.

Jack: Yeah, and I never loved . . . really . . . him. I still hate him. . . . He never let me love him. . . .

DLA: You may have to live with that sadness, but not with the hate.

Jack: Yeah . . . I want to stop hating. . . . He didn't know better.

. . . He had a rough childhood. . . . He was not educated. Just
rich and mean. . . .

DLA: I guess you are understanding why he was so bad.

Jack: . . . Yes, I don't have to hate him. . . .

DLA: To understand is to forgive.

Jack: Yes, I forgive him. . . . I'm so different from him. . . . He
never forgave anybody, ever. . . .

DLA: Look at your hate now.

Jack: It's not there now . . . just sadness . . . too bad! (long, intense silence) Very sad . . .

DLA: Your father hurt you, but you are rising above hate. This
will be your sadness for the rest of your life, but you can be
free of hate.

Jack: Yes, I don't hate him. . . . I forgive him . . . I'm sad that I
never had a father, but I forgive him. . . .

DLA: Stay with this for a little while longer, Jack. You are now
forgiving your father. You are freeing yourself from hatred.
You'll be free from hatred, but you'll always carry this sadness within you. Stay with this now.

Jack: (very relaxed and with a sad smile) . . . That's life, as Frank
Sinatra sings . . . that's life. Now everything is in place. Everything is clear. No foul smell anymore. . . . I have a good taste
in my mouth. . . . Yeah, very nice. . . . It sounds good, very
good. . . . Yeah.

DLA: I guess you have resolved this once and for all, Jack. Con-
gratulations! You are free to be yourself.

Jack: (still relaxed; a happier smile on his face now) Yes, I feel
light and happy . . . though sad too. It's strange, but I feel sad
and happy at the same time.

DLA: Then, Jack, go over it once more. You can be yourself. See
yourself as very different from your father. No hate. Just sadness . . . no need to be depressed anymore.

Jack: Yes, I'll be everything my father was not. (opening his eyes
and laughing) That'll show him, the bastard! He said it, remember, "I'm not stupid."

The session continued for a few minutes longer with our discussing what Jack had experienced. Since he did not want to

work on any other area of his life, we decided to discontinue
therapy but made a final appointment in six weeks' time, as a
follow-up.

Comments on the Third Session

Although Jack arrived in a good state of mind, the issue of his
feeling depressed since his father's death had not been resolved
yet. I reminded him of it and he agreed to work on it. This became
the goal for this session, completing the overall goal that he had
set for himself when seeking hypnotherapy. Jack was now able
to enter self-hypnosis quickly and smoothly. But, instead of being relaxed, he felt agitated. I led him into his agitation more fully
but emphasized awareness of bodily sensations ("What happens
in your body that you describe it as very agitated?"). He experienced an inner trembling all over his body which then turned
into sadness. When I invited him to become aware of any mental images that came up, I had in mind some materialization (see
Chapter 3) of his sadness: that he might perhaps experience his
sadness as a heavyweight on his chest or as a thick fog, for instance. But my expectation was not fulfilled. He regressed spontaneously to an important scene at the age of 10. This turned out
to be crucial and necessary in order for him to put his sadness
into perspective and to deal with the depression he had experienced following his father's death. His spontaneous regression
was announced by his change of voice, becoming childish. Join-
ing his regression I asked him questions in the present tense
("Where are you? What's your name? How old are you?") which
helped him to stay in his regressed experience. I called him Johnnie. While reporting the fight of his parents in the summer house,
his affect was that of a child, almost sobbing. It is interesting to
note that during this regression, he found himself lost in the dark,
outside the summer home, but later he was by the shack, no
longer lost and recognizing that part of the summer property.

The whole session proceeded in slow motion, with many
pauses, as indicated throughout the verbatim transcript. His
childish fear vanished quickly when he heard his mother calling

after him and he felt glad and happy. He was reassured by his mother, and protected from the fear of his father, once he let her discover him in his hiding place. Then, when the anxiety of the regression was resolved by reliving his mother's rescue, Jack came out of his self-hypnosis without any noticeable transition and quickly evaluated his "scene." In a mood of recollection he told me then the end of his parents relationship and about his mother's death. This led him back to his negative feelings about his father and, by going into them, he resolved his depression. It is amusing to note the transition from left- to right-hemispheric activity, and then back again, in his slip of the tongue ("Daddy— I'm sorry, I mean, a father"). But then, he let himself go into hypnosis once more and came up with the explanation for his depression. He still hoped to have a normal relationship with his father while he was alive and now there was no more hope left.

Even though consciously and logically he had denied it, subconsciously he did want to have a chance to love his father, a chance his father never provided for him. I personally felt his sadness and mentioned that he "may have to live with the sadness, not with the hate." This tapped his true desire to get rid of the hatred, and spontaneously drove him to a beautiful and quick enumeration of facts which helped him understand his father's nastiness and cruelty. Understanding may diminish hate and thus pave the way to forgiveness which, in Jack's case, was just ready to emerge, as his quick acceptance of my comment ("To understand is to forgive") indicated. Moreover, his forgiveness reinforced the conviction that he was not like his father ("I'm so different from him"). The resolution of his depression, which was the particular goal for this session, strengthened the overall goal for his hypnotherapy which was "not to be like his father." My comment about his rising above his father was geared to this same end.

I encouraged him to accept the sadness—*his* existential reality— of never having had a father in the emotional sense. Only when he was able to separate hate from sadness was the issue finished. The hatred, which he was able to dispel through forgiveness coming from understanding, freed him to be himself. By accepting the sadness of having been deprived of the love of a father and of his love for a father, he was able to go on with his life and enjoy it more fully.

It is extremely interesting to note how Jack closed this issue by using all his inner senses. The fact that he did this so spontaneously indicated to me a complete process of consolidation and resolution ("Now everything is in place"—kinetic sense; "everything is clear"—visual sense; "no foul smell any more"—olfactory sense; "I have a good taste in my mouth"—gustatory sense; "it sounds good"—hearing sense). And it should be noted that Jack was not psychologically sophisticated or well-read. This process really came from an experiential level, the way he was integrating this issue subconsciously.

CONCLUSION

The follow-up session, which lasted only about half an hour, indicated that the gains obtained in the three hypnotherapy sessions had lasted. Moreover, it showed a generalization of results, both in his personal and occupational life. Jack was very pleased with what he had accomplished in hypnotherapy and stated that his whole life was more relaxed and enjoyable. He had even become more productive and ambitious, hoping to get a much better job, for which he had been interviewed three days before the follow-up session. He laughed, saying that he was going to end up like his father, after all. He also reported that his relationship with his lady was better than ever and that he had taught her relaxation and self-hypnosis, a practice both now enjoyed frequently. Because Jack had come to hypnotherapy to work on a specific problem and it had been resolved, the therapeutic relationship was terminated.

The learned reader may speculate on the course this clinical case could have taken if more traditional forms of nonhypnotic, talk therapy had been followed. But this is not the place for comparisons. I merely hope that the detailed description of the two cases presented in this and the previous chapter will help those with "a beginner's mind" (as was mentioned in Chapter 5) to consider the merits of this approach to human transformation—to metanoia.

Epilogue

One of my grandfathers, José León Suárez, was a famous man in Argentina. There is a town near Buenos Aires and a street in the capital of the country named after him. He was a writer, an intellectual, a political scientist, and a diplomat. I grew up having him as my model, though he died before my birth. I wanted to be, like my grandfather, a famous man, respected for his writing. But then, as years went by, I found myself fearing that the moment I finished my first book I would die. Since my superstitious prophecy was not fulfilled, I felt better about writing this present volume. Another factor that influenced me was the encouragement I received from all the book reviews of *Hypnosis and Sex Therapy* and from the many organizations that asked me to either talk or lead seminars on that subject matter. In that book I had a chapter on the New Hypnosis. At the request of several people whose minds I respect and admire, I set out to elaborate and clarify the concept of the New Hypnosis more fully. Once I started, I realized that much more than I was ready to put down on paper could be written about it. The task was to select the main ideas and issues and to try to present them with clarity and a sense of clinical applicability.

My attempt has been to provide a practical view of hypnosis as a valuable clinical method. My hope is that only readers with a "beginner's mind" will plow through the pages of this book. My joy will be to know that "the Doctors of the soul" will find in it means to make their work more effective. The people who trust us, psychotherapists, demand much from us but deserve the best we can give them. Although I started in a strict psychoanalytical mode, thanks to the influence of several great teachers including Erich Fromm, I dared to test less ''orthodox'' approaches in psychotherapy. Having gone through a wide range of methods and theoretical schools, I finally found that the approach I have tried to present in this book is most effective, most elegant, and most respectful to clients. Having practiced it for over seven years, I thought it was time to outline it in a book.

Some points in my presentation will be questioned and debated. I believe that controversy is the necessary vehicle to reach new heights of knowledge, because controversy, if respectful, leads to further investigation and research, which, in turn, leads to new evidence. I am fortunate that this book is being published at a time when the public as well as the professional community is receptive to the idea of subconscious processes, of the importance of one's inner experience, of the value of right-hemispheric thinking (as I have called it throughout the book, oversimplifying, for didactic purposes, processes that are still being investigated and far from definitively known). The constant attention to the inner processes and experiences of clients has led me to the conviction that the so-called scientific method of investigation is far from adequate for research. I am lucky that serious intellectuals in our own field (see Lieberman, 1977) have questioned the experimental method more adequately than I could ever do.

This book was written in a difficult period in my life, while I was going through important personal and family changes, with all the hurt, confusion, and illusions that such circumstances bring. Writing became difficult and painful many times. It was done while battling my own demons. Often they stopped the writing altogether. The encouragement of many people mentioned in the Acknowledgments, and especially of Bernie Mazel and Ann Alhadeff of Brunner/Mazel Publishers, made the completion of this book possible.

The New Hypnosis is a personal toast to shattered dreams and to new rainbows. It is the revelation of my work and my professional legacy. Although "there is nothing new under the sun," the new built on the old has the power to enrich. *The New Hypnosis* tries to show that possibility of enrichment for those whose task is to help others go through the process of metanoia.

References

Ader, R. (Ed.). *Psychoneuroimmunology*. New York: Academic Press, 1981.

American Society of Clinical Hypnosis. *Syllabus of Hypnosis*. Des Plains, IL: American Society of Clinical Hypnosis, 1973.

Applebaum, S. A. A psychoanalyst looks at Gestalt therapy. In C. Hatcher & P. Himelstein (Eds.), *The Handbook of Gestalt Therapy*. New York: Jason Aronson, 1976.

Araoz, D. L. Clinical hypnosis in couple therapy. *The Journal of the American Society of Psychosomatic Dentistry and Medicine*, 1978, 25(2), 58–67.

Araoz, D. L. Hypnosis in couples group counseling. Paper presented to the American Psychological Association Meeting, New York, 1979.

Araoz, D. L. Negative self-hypnosis. *Journal of Contemporary Psychotherapy*, 1981, 12(1), 45–51.

Araoz, D. L. *Hypnosis and Sex Therapy*. New York: Brunner/Mazel, 1982. (a).

Araoz, D. L. The New Hypnosis. Paper presented to the 25th Annual Scientific Meeting, American Society of Clinical Hypnosis, Denver, CO, 1982. (b).

Araoz, D. L. The paradox of the New Hypnosis. Paper presented at the meeting of the American Society of Clinical Hypnosis, Dallas, TX, November, 1983.

Araoz, D. L. The New Hypnosis: The quintessence of client-centeredness. In J. K. Zeig (Ed.), *Ericksonian Psychotherapy. Vol. 1: Structures*. New York: Brunner/Mazel, 1985.

Araoz, D. L. Use of hypnotic techniques with oncology patients. *Journal of Psychosocial Oncology*, 1984, 1(4), 47–54. (a).

Araoz, D. L. Hypnosis in management training and development. In W. C. Wester, II & A. H. Smith (Eds.), *Clinical Hypnosis: A Multidisciplinary Approach*. Philadelphia, PA: Lippincott, 1984. (b).

Araoz, D. L. Hypnosex therapy: What if it is more than just about sexual functioning? Presentation to the International Society of Professional Hypnosis, New York, 1984. (c).

Araoz, D. L., & Bleck, R. T. *Hypnosex*. New York: Arbor House, 1982.

Barber, J. Hypnosis and the unhypnotizable. *American Journal of Clinical Hypnosis*, 1980, 23, 4–9.

197

Barber, J. Incorporating hypnosis in the management of chronic pain. In J. Barber & C. Adrian (Eds.), *Psychological Approaches to the Management of Pain*. New York: Brunner/Mazel, 1982.

Barber, J., & Adrian, C. *Psychological Approaches to the Management of Pain*. New York: Brunner/Mazel, 1982.

Barber, T. X. Hypnosis as perceptual-cognitive restructuring: III. From somnambulism to autohypnosis. *Journal of Psychology*, 1957, 44, 299–304.

Barber, T. X. *Hypnosis: A Scientific Approach*. New York: Van Nostrand Reinhold, 1969. (Reprinted in 1981 by Powers Publishers, 60 Vose, South Orange, NJ).

Barber, T. X. *LSD, Marihuana, Yoga and Hypnosis*. Hawthorne, NY: Aldine, 1970.

Barber, T. X. Suggested "hypnotic" behavior: The trance paradigm vs. an alternative paradigm. In E. Fromm & R. E. Shor (Eds.), *Hypnosis: Research Developments and Perspectives*. Chicago, IL: Aldine, 1972.

Barber, T. X. *Hypnosis and Psychosomatics*. San Francisco, CA: Proseminar Institute, 1978.

Barber, T. X. Training students to use self-suggestions for personal growth: Methods and word-by-word instructions. *Journal of Suggestive-Accelerative Learning and Teaching*, 1979, 4(2), 111–128. (a).

Barber, T. X. Eidetic imagery and the ability to hallucinate at will. *Behavioral and Brain Sciences*, 1979, 2, 596–597. (b).

Barber, T. X. Innovations and limitations in Erickson's hypnosis. *Contemporary Psychology*, 1981, 26(11), 825–827. (a).

Barber, T. X. Medicine, suggestive therapy and healing. In R. J. Kastenbaum, T. X. Barber, S. C. Wilson, B. L. Ryder, & L. B. Hathaway (Eds.), *Old, Sick and Helpless: Where Therapy Begins*. Cambridge, MA: Ballinger, 1981. (b).

Barber, T. X. Hypnosuggestive procedures in the treatment of clinical pain: Implications for theories of hypnosis and suggestive therapy. In T. Millon, C. Green, & R. Meagher (Eds.), *Handbook of Clinical Health Psychology*. New York: Plenum Press, 1982, 521–560. (a).

Barber, T. X. Eidetic imagery as very vivid imagery and as hallucinatory behavior. *Journal of Mental Imagery*, 1982, 6(1), 32–35. (b).

Barber, T. X. *Hypnosuggestive techniques*. (Two-day professional training program). Evaluation Research Associates. Syracuse, NY: 1983.

Barber, T. X. Changing "unchangeable" bodily processes by (hypnotic) suggestions: A new look at hypnosis, cognitions, imaginings and the mind-body problem. In A. A. Sheikh (Ed.), *Imagination and Healing*. Farmingdale, NY: Baywood, 1984. (a).

Barber, T. X. Hypnosis, deep relaxation and active relaxation: Data, theory and clinical applications. In P. Lehrer & R. Woolfolk (Eds.), *Principles and Practice of Stress Management*. New York: Guilford Press, 1984. (b).

Barber, T. X. Hypnosuggestive procedures as catalysts for all psychotherapies. In S. Lynn & J. P. Garske (Eds.), *Contemporary Psychotherapies: Models and Methods*. Columbus, OH: Charles E. Merrill, in press.

Barber, T. X., Spanos, N. P., & Chaves, J. F. *Hypnotism: Imagination and Human Potentialities*. New York: Pergamon, 1974.

Barber, T. X., & Wilson, S. C. Hypnosis, suggestions and altered states of consciousness: Experimental evaluation of the new cognitive-behavioral theory and the traditional trance-state theory of "hypnosis." *Annals of the New York Academy of Sciences*, 1977, 296, 34–47.

Barber, T. X., & Wilson, S. C. The Barber Suggestibility Scale and the Creative Imagination Scale: Experimental and clinical applications. *American Journal of Clinical Hypnosis*, 1979, 21, 83–108.

Barrett-Lennard, G. Dimensions of perceived therapist response related to therapeutic change. Doctoral dissertation, University of Chicago, 1959.

Baudouin, C. *Suggestion and Autosuggestion*. New York: Dodd, Mead, 1922.

Beck, A. T. *Cognitive Therapy and the Emotional Disorders*. New York: International Universities Press, 1976.

Beisser, A. R. The paradoxical theory of change. In J. Fagan & J. L. Shepherd (Eds.), *Gestalt Therapy Now*. Palo Alto, CA: Science and Behavior Books, 1970.

Bennett, H. Z. *The Doctor Within*. New York: Clarkson N. Potter, 1981.

Benson, H., & Epstein, M. D. The placebo effect: A neglected asset in the care of patients. *Journal of the American Medical Association*, 1975, 232, 1225–1227.

Bernheim, H. M. *Hypnosis and Suggestion in Psychotherapy: A Treatise on the Nature and Uses of Hypnotism*. (English translation, 1888, reissued by E. R. Hilgard). New Hyde Park, NY: University Books, 1964.

Blumenthal, R. A. Rational suggestion therapy: A subconscious approach to RET. *Medical Hypnoanalysis*, 1984, 5(2), 57–60.

Boszormenyi-Nagy, I. The concept of change in family therapy. In A. Friedman (Ed.), *Psychotherapy for the Whole Family*. New York: Springer, 1965.

Bowers, K. S. Hypnosis: An informational approach. *Annals of the New York Academy of Sciences*, 1977, 206, 222–237.

Bowers, K. S., & Kelly, P. Stress, disease, psychotherapy and hypnosis. *Journal of Abnormal Psychology*, 1979, 85(5), 490–505.

Boy, A. V., & Pine, G. J. *Client-centered Counseling: A Renewal*. Boston: Allyn & Bacon, 1982.

Braun, B. G. Family therapy with hypnosis. Unpublished paper. Chicago, IL: Associated Mental Health Services, 1978.

Braun, B. G. Hypnosis in family therapy. In W. C. Wester, II & A. H. Smith (Eds.), *Clinical Hypnosis: A Multidisciplinary Approach*. Philadelphia, PA: Lippincott, 1984.

Bresler, D. *Free Yourself from Pain*. New York: Simon & Schuster, 1977.

Calof, D. Hypnosis in marital therapy: Toward a transgenerational approach. In J. K. Zeig (Ed.), *Ericksonian Psychotherapy. Vol. II: Clinical Applications*. New York: Brunner/Mazel, 1985.

Coe, W. C., & Ryken, K. Hypnosis and risk to human subjects. *American Psychologist*, 1979, 34, 673–681.

Coe, W. C., & Sharcoff, J. An empirical evaluation of the Neurolinguistic Programming model. Paper presented at the annual meeting of the American Psychological Association, Anaheim, CA, 1983.

Dammann, C. Family therapy. Paper presented at the 2nd International Congress of Ericksonian Approaches to Hypnosis and Psychotherapy, Phoenix, AZ, 1983.

De Stefano, R. The "inoculation" effect in think-with instructions for "hypnotic-like" experiences. Doctoral dissertation, Temple University, 1977.

Diamond, M. J. The use of observationally-presented information to modify hypnotic susceptibility. *Journal of Abnormal Psychology*, 1972, 79, 174–180.

Diamond, M. J. Modification of hypnotizability: A review. *Psychological Bulletin*, 1974, 81, 180–198.

Diamond, M. J. Hypnotizability is modifiable: An alternative approach. *International Journal of Clinical and Experimental Hypnosis*, 1977, 25, 147–166. (a).

Diamond, M. J. Issues and methods for modifying responsivity to hypnosis. *Annals of the New York Academy of Sciences*, 1977, 296, 199–228. (b).

Diamond, M. J. Clinical hypnosis: Towards a cognitive-based skill approach. Paper presented at the annual meeting of the American Psychological Association, Toronto, 1978.

Diamond, M. J. The client-as-hypnotist: Furthering hypnotherapeutic change. *International Journal of Clinical and Experimental Hypnosis*, 1980, 28, 197–207.

Diamond, M. J. It takes two to tango: Some thoughts on the neglected importance of the hypnotist in an interactive hypnotherapeutic relationship. Paper presented at the Annual Scientific Meeting, American Society of Clinical Hypnosis, Denver, CO, 1982. (a).

Diamond, M. J. Modifying hypnotic experience by means of indirect hypnosis and hypnotic skill training: An update (1981). *Research Communications in Psychology, Psychiatry and Behavior*, 1982, 7, 233–239. (b).

Diamond, M. J. Reflections on the interactive nature of the hypnotic experience: On the relational dimensions of hypnosis. Presidential address, Division of Psychological Hypnosis of the American Psychological Association, Anaheim, CA, 1983. (a).

Diamond, M. J. The cognitive skills model: An emerging paradigm for investigating hypnotic phenomena. Unpublished manuscript, 1983. (b).

Edelstien, M. G. *Trauma, Trance and Transformation: A Clinical Guide to Hypnotherapy*. New York: Brunner/Mazel, 1981.

Einstein, A. Ether and the theory of relativity. In W. Perret & G. B. Jeffrey (Eds.), *Side Lights on Relativity*. London: Methuen, 1922.

Einstein, A., & Infeld, L. *The Evolution of Physics*. New York: Simon & Schuster, 1961.

Ellis, A. *Humanistic Psychotherapy*. New York: McGraw-Hill, 1973.

Engel, G. L. Sudden and rapid death during psychological stress: Folklore or folk wisdom? *Annals of Internal Medicine*, 1971, 74, 771–782.

Erickson, M. H. A study of an experimental neurosis hypnotically induced in a case of ejaculatio precox. *British Journal of Medical Psychology*, 1935, 15, 34–50.

Erickson, M. H., & Rossi, E. L. Varieties of double bind. *American Journal of Clinical Hypnosis*, 1975, 17, 143–157.

Erickson, M. H., & Rossi, E. L. *Hypnotherapy: An Exploratory Casebook*. New York: Irvington, 1979.

Erickson, M. H., & Rossi, E. L. *Experiencing Hypnosis*. New York: Irvington, 1981.

Erickson, M. H., Rossi, E. L., & Rossi, S. *Hypnotic Realities*. New York: Irvington, 1976.

Evans-Wentz, W. Y. (1927). *The Tibetan Book of the Dead*. New York: Oxford University Press, 1960.

Eysenck, H. J. *The Biological Basis of Personality*. Springfield, IL: Charles C Thomas, 1967.

Field, P. B. Humanistic aspects of hypnotic communication. In E. Fromm & R. E. Shor (Eds.), *Hypnosis: Developments in Research and New Perspectives* (2nd Edition). Hawthorne, NY: Aldine, 1979.

Finkelstein, S., & Howard, M. G. Cancer prevention—A three year pilot study. *American Journal of Clinical Hypnosis*, 1983, (2–3), 177–183.

Flavell, J. H. *The Developmental Psychology of Jean Piaget*. New York: Van Nostrand, 1963.

Ford, D. H., & Urban, B. H. *Systems of Psychotherapy*. New York: Wiley, 1965.

Framo, J. *Family Interaction: A Dialogue Between Family Researchers and Family Therapists*. New York: Springer, 1972.

Fromm, E. An ego-psychological theory of altered states of consciousness. *International Journal of Clinical and Experimental Hypnosis*, 1977, 25, 372–387.

Fromm, E., Brown, D. P., Hurt, S. W., Oberlander, J. Z., Boxer, A. M., & Pheiffer, G. The phenomena and characteristics of self-hypnosis. *International Journal of Clinical and Experimental Hypnosis*, 1981, 29, 189–246.

Gendlin, E. *Focusing*. New York: Everest House, 1978.

Gibson, H. B. Book review of E. L. Rossi (Ed.), *The Collected Papers of Milton H. Erickson on Hypnosis* (Vols. I & II). New York: Irvington, 1980. *International Journal of Clinical and Experimental Hypnosis*, 1984, 32(2), 254–256.

Gill, M. M., & Brenman, M. *Hypnosis and Related States*. New York: International Universities Press, 1959.

Goba, H. K. Hypnosis in marriage counseling. Paper presented at the annual meeting of the American Society of Clinical Hypnosis, St. Louis, MO, 1978.

Goba, H. K. Guided self-hypnosis. In G. D. Burrows, D. R. Collison, & L. Dennerstein (Eds.), *Hypnosis 1979*. New York: Elsevier North-Holland Biomedical Press, 1979.

Goba, H. K. *Your Thoughts and You*. Calgary: H. K. Goba, 1983.

Gordon, D. *Therapeutic Metaphors*. Cupertino, CA: Meta Publications, 1978.

Gross, M. Aspects of self-hypnosis. *Medical Hypnoanalysis*, 1984, 6(2), 75–79.

Haley, J. (Ed.). *Advanced Techniques of Hypnosis and Therapy: Selected Papers of M. H. Erickson*. New York: Grune & Stratton, 1967.

Haley, J. *Uncommon Therapy: The Psychiatric Techniques of M. H. Erickson*. New York: Norton, 1973.

Haley, J. *Problem-Solving Therapy*. San Francisco, CA: Jossey-Bass, 1976.

Halkides, G. An experimental study of four conditions necessary for therapeutic personality change. Doctoral dissertation, University of Chicago, 1958.

Hall, H. R. Hypnosis and the immune system: A review with implications for cancer and the psychology of healing. *American Journal of Clinical Hypnosis*, 1983, 25(2–3), 92–103.

Hall, H. R. Imagery and cancer. In A. A. Sheikh (Ed.), *Imagination and Healing*. Farmingdale, NY: Baywood, 1984.

Hart, J. T., & Tomlison, T. M. (Eds.). *New Directions in Client-centered Therapy*. Boston, MA: Houghton Mifflin, 1970.

Hilgard, E. R. *Divided Consciousness: Multiple Controls in Human Thought and Action*. New York: Wiley, 1977.

Hilgard, E. R., & Hilgard, J. R. *Hypnosis in the Relief of Pain*. Los Altos, CA: William Kaufman, 1975.

Holden, C. Cancer and the mind: How they are connected. *Science*, 1978, 200, 1363–1369.

Hunt, M. Self-hypnosis works. *The Reader's Digest*, April 1984, 164–169.

Ikemi, Y., & Ikemi, A. Psychosomatic medicine: A meeting ground of Eastern and Western medicine. *Journal of the American Society of Psychosomatic Den-*

tistry and Medicine, 1983, 30, 3–16.

Illich, I. *Medical Nemesis*. New York: Pantheon, 1976.

Jaffe, D. T. *Healing From Within*. New York: Bantam Books, 1980.

Kaplan, H. S. *The New Sex Therapy*. New York: Brunner/Mazel, 1976.

Katz, N. W. Hypnotic inductions as training in cognitive self-control. *Cognitive Therapy and Research*, 1978, 2, 365–369.

Katz, N. W. Increasing hypnotic responsiveness: Behavioral training vs. trance induction. *Journal of Consulting and Clinical Psychology*, 1979, 47(1), 119–127.

Katz, N. W., & Crawford, V. L. A little trance and a little skill: Interaction between models of hypnosis and type of hypnotic induction. Paper presented at the annual meeting of the Society for Clinical and Experimental Hypnosis, Ashville, NC, 1978.

Kinney, J. M., & Sachs, L. B. Increasing hypnotic susceptibility. *Journal of Abnormal Psychology*, 1974, 83, 145–150.

Kleinman, A., Eisenberg, L., & Good, B. Culture, illness and care: Clinical lessons from anthropologic and cross-cultural research. *Annals of Internal Medicine*, 1978, 88(2), 251–258.

Kramer, C. (Ed.). The theoretical position: Diagnostic and therapeutic implications. In *Beginning Phase of Family Treatment*. Chicago, IL: Kramer Foundation, 1968.

Kris, E. *Psychoanalytic Explorations in Art*. New York: International Universities Press, 1952. (Original publication, 1934).

Kroger, W. S., & Fezler, W. D. *Hypnosis and Behavior Modification: Imagery Conditioning*. Philadelphia, PA: Lippincott, 1976.

Krumboltz, J. D. *Behavior Therapy or Client-centered Therapy* (A debate with C. H. Patterson). Film, American Personnel and Guidance Association, 1979.

Kuhner, A. Hypnosis without hypnosis. *International Journal of Clinical and Experimental Hypnosis*, 1962, 10, 93–99.

Lankton, S. R. Multiple-embedded metaphor and diagnosis. In J. K. Zeig (Ed.), *Ericksonian Psychotherapy. Vol 1: Structures*. New York: Brunner/Mazel, 1985.

Lankton, S. R., & Lankton, C. H. Indirect suggestions and binds in family therapy. (Workshop handout). *Ericksonian Approaches to Psychotherapy*. Gulf Breeze, FL: Lankton, 1982.

Lankton, S. R., & Lankton, C. H. *The Answer Within: A Clinical Framework of Ericksonian Hypnotherapy*. New York: Brunner/Mazel, 1983.

Levi-Strauss, C. *Structural Anthropology*. New York: Basic Books, 1963.

Levitsky, A., & Simkin, J. S. Gestalt therapy. In L. N. Solomon & B. Berzon (Eds.), *New Perspectives on Encounter Groups*. San Francisco, CA: Jossey-Bass, 1972.

Ley, R. G., & Freeman, R. J. Imagery, cerebral laterality and the healing process. In A. A. Sheikh (Ed.), *Imagination and Healing*. Farmingdale, NY: Baywood, 1984.

Lieberman, L. R. Hypnosis research and the limitations of the experimental method. *Annals of the New York Academy of Sciences*, 1977, 296, 60–68.

Loriedo, C. Tailoring suggestions in family therapy. In J. K. Zeig (Ed.), *Ericksonian Psychotherapy. Vol II: Clinical Applications*. New York: Brunner/Mazel, 1985.

Lovern, J. D., & Zohn, J. Utilization and indirect suggestion in multiple family group therapy with alcoholics. *Journal of Marital and Family Therapy*, 1982, 8, 325–333.

Lynch, J. J. *The Broken Heart: The Medical Consequences of Loneliness*. New York: Basic Books, 1977.

Madanes, C. *Strategic Family Therapy*. San Francisco, CA: Jossey-Bass, 1981.

Mahrer, A. R. *Experiential Psychotherapy: Basic Practices*. New York: Brunner/ Mazel, 1983.

Maturana, H. *Biology of Cognition* (Report A.O.). Urbana, IL: Biological Computer Laboratory, 1970.

May, R. Contributions of existential psychotherapy. In R. May, E. Angel, & H. F. Ellenberger (Eds.), *Existence: A New Dimension in Psychiatry and Psychology*. New York: Basic Books, 1958.

Mazza, J. Family therapy. Paper presented at the 2nd International Congress of Ericksonian Approaches to Hypnosis and Psychotherapy, Phoenix, AZ, 1983.

McMahon, C. E. The role of imagination in the disease process: Pre-Cartesian history. *Psychological Medicine*, 1976, 6, 179–184.

Meador, B. D., & Rogers, C. R. Person-centered therapy. In R. J. Corsini (Ed.), *Current Psychotherapies* (2nd edition). Itasca, IL: F. E. Peacock, 1979.

Mears, A. Mind and cancer. *Lancet*, 1979, 8123, 978.

Meichenbaum, D. *Cognitive Behavior Modification*. Morristown, NJ: General Learning Press, 1974.

Miller, G. A., Galanter, E., & Pribram, K. H. *Plans and the Structure of Behavior*. New York: Holt, Rinehart & Winston, 1960.

Miller, H. Process therapy. Paper presented at the meeting of the American Society of Clinical Hypnosis, Boston, MA, 1981.

Minuchin, S. *Families and Family Therapy*. Cambridge, MA: Harvard University Press, 1974.

Minuchin, S., Baker, L., & Rosman, B. *Psychosomatic Families*. Cambridge, MA: Harvard University Press, 1978.

Morris, G. O., & Gardner, C. W. Contributions to the theory of the hypnotic process and the established hypnotic state. *Psychiatry*, 1959, 22, 377–398.

Morrison, J. K. The use of imagery techniques in Family Therapy. *American Journal of Family Therapy*, 1981, 9(22), 52–56.

M'Uzan, M. de. Psychodynamic mechanism in psychosomatic symptom formation. *Psychotherapy and Psychosomatics*, 1974, 23, 103–110.

Naranjo, C. *The Unfolding of Man*. Menlo Park, CA: Stanford Research Institute, 1969.

Nunberg, H. *Practice and Theory of Psychoanalysis*. New York: Nervous and Mental Disease Monographs, 1948.

Oyle, I. *The Healing Mind*. New York: Pocket Books, 1976.

Pelletier, K. *Mind as Healer, Mind as Slayer*. New York: Delta, 1979.

Perls, F. Gestalt therapy verbatim: Introduction. In C. Hatcher & P. Himelstein (Eds.), *The Handbook of Gestalt Therapy*. New York: Jason Aronson, 1976.

Perls, L. Some aspects of Gestalt therapy. Paper presented at the annual meeting of the American Orthopsychiatric Association, New York, 1973.

Polanyi, M. *Personal Knowledge: Toward a Postcritical Philosophy*. New York: Harper & Row, 1964.

Popper, K. R. *Unended Quest.* La Salle, IL: Open Court, 1974.

Pribram, K. *Languages of the Brain: Experimental Paradoxes and Principles in Neuropsychology.* Monterey, CA: Brooks/Cole, 1971.

Remen, N. *The Human Patient.* New York: Doubleday, 1980.

Ritterman, M. *Using Hypnosis in Family Therapy.* San Francisco, CA: Jossey-Bass, 1983.

Rogers, C. R. A theory of therapy, personality and interpersonal relationships as developed in the client-centered framework. In S. Koch (Ed.), *Psychology: A Study of a Science, Vol. III, Formulations of the Person and the Social Context.* New York: McGraw-Hill, 1959.

Rogers, C. R. *On Becoming a Person.* Boston, MA: Houghton Mifflin, 1961.

Rogers, C. R., Gendlin, E. T., Kiesler, D. J., & Louax, C. (Eds.). *The Therapeutic Relationship and Its Impact: A Study of Psychotherapy With Schizophrenics.* Madison, WI: University of Wisconsin Press, 1967.

Rosenthal, R., & Jacobson, L. *Pygmalion in the Classroom: Teacher Expectation and Pupils' Intellectual Ability.* New York: Holt, Rinehart & Winston, 1968.

Rossi, E. L. The cerebral hemispheres in analytical psychology. *Journal of Analytical Psychology,* 1977, 22, 32–51.

Rossi, E. L. (Ed.). *The Collected Papers of Milton H. Erickson on Hypnosis* (4 vols.). New York: Irvington, 1980.

Sacerdote, P. Teaching self-hypnosis to adults. *International Journal of Clinical and Experimental Hypnosis,* 1981, 29, 282–299.

Sachs, L. B., & Anderson, W. L. Modification of hypnotic susceptibility. *International Journal of Clinical and Experimental Hypnosis,* 1967, 15, 172–180.

Samuels, M., & Bennett, H. Z. *Spirit Guides.* New York: Random House/Bookwords, 1974.

Sarbin, T. R. Contributions to role-taking theory: 1. Hypnotic behavior. *Psychological Review,* 1950, 57, 255–270.

Sarbin, T. R. Attempts to understand hypnotic phenomena. In L. Postman (Ed.), *Psychology in the Making: History of Selected Research Problems.* New York: Knopf, 1962.

Sarbin, T. R., & Andersen, M. L. Role-theoretical analysis of hypnotic behavior. In J. E. Gordon (Ed.), *Handbook of Clinical and Experimental Hypnosis.* New York: Macmillan, 1967.

Sarbin, T. R., & Coe, W. C. *Hypnosis: A Social Psychological Analysis of Influence Communication.* New York: Macmillan, 1972.

Schleifer, S. J., Keller, S. E., McKegney, F. P., & Stein, M. Bereavement and lymphocyte function. Paper presented at the annual meeting of the American Psychiatric Association, San Francisco, CA, 1980.

Selvini Palazzoli, M. Why a long interval between sessions? In M. Andolfi & I. Zwerling (Eds.), *Dimensions of Family Therapy.* New York: Guilford Press, 1980.

Selvini Palazzoli, M., Boscolo, L., Cecchin, G., & Prata, G. *Paradox and Counterparadox.* New York: Jason Aronson, 1978.

Selye, H. *Stress in Health and Disease.* Reading, MA: Butterworths, 1976.

Shames, R., & Sterin, C. *Healing with Mind Power.* Emmaus, PA: Rodale Press, 1978.

Shaw, L. H. *Hypnosis in Practice.* London: Baillière Tindall, 1977.

Sheikh, A. A. (Ed.). *Imagery: Current Theory, Research and Applications*. New York: Wiley, 1982.

Sheikh, A. A., Richardson, P., & Moleski, L. M. Psychosomatics and mental imagery. In A. A. Sheikh & J. T. Shaffer (Eds.), *The Potential of Fantasy and Imagination*. New York: Brandon House, 1979.

Sheikh, A. A., & Shaffer, J. T. (Eds.). *The Potential of Fantasy and Imagination*. New York: Brandon House, 1979.

Shekelle, R. B., Raynor, Jr., W. J., Ostfeld,, A. M., Garron, D. C., Bieliauskas, L. A., Liu, S. C., Maliza, C., & Oglesby, P. Psychological depression and 17-year-old risk of death from cancer. *Psychosomatic Medicine*, 1981, 43, 117–125.

Shertzer, B., & Stone, S. C. *Fundamentals of Counseling* (2nd edition). Boston, MA: Houghton Mifflin, 1974.

Shor, R. E. Hypnosis and the concept of the generalized reality-orientation. *American Journal of Psychotherapy*, 1959, 13, 582–602.

Shulik, A. M. Right- vs. left-hemispheric communication styles in hypnotic inductions and the facilitation of hypnotic trance. Doctoral dissertation, California School of Professional Psychology. San Francisco, CA, 1979.

Simkin, J. S. Gestalt therapy. In R. J. Corsini (Ed.), *Current Psychotherapies* (2nd edition). Itasca, IL: F. E. Peacock, 1979.

Singer, J. L. *The Inner World of Daydreaming*. New York: Harper & Row, 1975.

Singer, J. L., & Pope, K. S. (Eds.). *The Power of Human Imagination*. New York: Plenum Press, 1978.

Spanos, N. P. Goal-directed fantasy and the performance of hypnotic test suggestions. *Psychiatry*, 1971, 34, 86–96.

Spiegel, H. *Manual for Hypnotic Induction Profile: Eye Roll Levitation Method* (revised edition). New York: Soni Medica, 1973.

Stuart, R. B. *Trick or Treatment: How and When Psychotherapy Fails*. Champaign, IL: Research Press, 1970.

Sullivan, H. S. *The Interpersonal Theory of Psychiatry*. New York: Norton, 1953.

Suzuki, S. *Zen Mind, Beginner's Mind*. New York: Weatherhill, 1970.

Szent-Gyoergyi. Drive in living matter to perfect itself. *Synthesis*, 1974, 1(1), 12–24.

Tart, C. T. Quick and convenient assessment of hypnotic depth: Self-report scales. *American Journal of Clinical Hypnosis*, 1979, 21, 186–207.

Tossi, D. J., Reardon, J. P., & Rudy, D. Cognitive experiential therapy. Paper presented at the annual meeting of the American Society of Clinical Hypnosis, Atlanta, GA, 1977.

Truax, C. B., & Carkhuff, R. R. *Towards Effective Counseling and Psychotherapy: Training and Practice*. Chicago, IL: Aldine, 1967.

Truax, C. B., & Mitchell, K. M. Research on certain therapist interpersonal skills in relation to process outcome. In A. E. Bergin & J. L. Garfield (Eds.), *Handbook of Psychotherapy and Behavior Change*. New York: Wiley, 1971.

Watkins, J. G. The affect bridge: A hypnoanalytic technique. *International Journal of Clinical and Experimental Hypnosis*, January 1971, 19, 21–27.

Watkins, J. G. *The Therapeutic Self*. New York: Human Sciences Press, 1978.

Watzlawick, P. *How Real is Real? Confusion, Disinformation, Communication*. New York: Random House, 1976.

Watzlawick, P. *The Language of Change*. New York: Basic Books, 1978.
Watzlawick, P. Erickson's contribution to the interactional view of psychotherapy. In J. K. Zeig (Ed.), *Ericksonian Approaches to Hypnosis and Psychotherapy*. New York: Brunner/Mazel, 1982.
Watzlawick, P. (Ed.) *The Invented Reality*. New York: Norton, 1984.
Watzlawick, P. Hypnotherapy without trance. In J. K. Zeig (Ed.), *Ericksonian Psychotherapy. Vol. I: Structures*. New York: Brunner/Mazel, 1985.
Watzlawick, P., Weakland, J., & Fisch, R. *Change: Principles of Problem Formation and Problem Resolution*. New York: Norton, 1974.
Weeks, G. R., & L'Abate, L. *Paradoxical Psychotherapy*. New York: Brunner/ Mazel, 1982.
Weinstock, C. Further evidence on psychobiological aspects of cancer. *International Journal of Psychosomatics*, 1984, 31(1), 20–22.
Weitzenhoffer, A. M. *General Techniques of Hypnotism*. New York: Grune & Stratton, 1957.
Weitzenhoffer, A. M., & Hilgard, E. R. *Stanford Hypnotic Susceptibility Scale, Forms A and B*. Palo Alto, CA: Consulting Psychologists Press, 1959.
Weitzenhoffer, A. M., & Hilgard, E. R. *Stanford Hypnotic Susceptibility Scale, Form C*. Palo Alto, CA: Consulting Psychologists Press, 1962.
Wick, E. Unification of hypnosis theories. Paper presented to the annual meeting of the New York Society of Clinical Hypnosis, New York, 1983.
Wilson, S. C., & Barber, T. X. The Creative Imagination Scale as a measure of hypnotic responsiveness. *American Journal of Clinical Hypnosis*, 1978, 20, 235–249.
Wilson, S. C., & Barber, T. X. The fantasy-prone personality: Implications for understanding imagery, hypnosis and parapsychological phenomena. In A. A. Sheikh (Ed.), *Imagery: Current Theory, Research and Applications*. New York: Wiley, 1982.
Wolberg, L. R. *Hypnoanalysis*. New York: Grune & Stratton, 1964.
Yalom, I. D. *Existential Psychotherapy*. New York: Basic Books, 1980.
Zeig, J. (Ed.). *Ericksonian Approaches to Hypnosis and Psychotherapy*. New York: Brunner/Mazel, 1982.
Zeig, J. (Ed.). *Ericksonian Psychotherapy. Vol. II: Clinical Applications*. New York: Brunner/Mazel, 1985.
Zilbergeld, B. *The Shrinking of America*. Boston, MA: Little, Brown, 1983.
Zukav, G. *The Dancing Wu Li Masters*. New York: Bantam Books, 1979.

Name Index

Subject Index